Introduction

The occupational therapist must offer a unique and focused contribution to the health care of psychosocially dysfunctional people. This requires some consensus about what the field's unique role is. While many occupational therapists do experience ambiguity over the nature of their service, this need not be the case. Occupational therapy has a rich and long history that readily yields a vision of therapists' roles and functions in the psychosocial arena. The purpose of this book is to identify the role and mission of occupational therapy, beginning two centuries ago as moral treatment and continuing today in the use of occupation as a psychosocial health determinant. These principles and practices are unique and contribute substantially to the care of psychosocially dysfunctional people.

Those with a clear identity and commitment to their own professional perspective can more effectively contribute to the function of the team and to patient care. Those who lack clarity and conviction about their professional role identity more often blend into the setting, becoming ancillary to others with stronger perspectives. They tend to follow rather than to direct and develop the goals and activities of the settings in which they practice. This was borne out in a nationwide study of psychosocial occupational therapists.* Therapists who reported that they used activities for psychodynamic reasons (e.g., patients working with clay in order to ventilate anger) generally did so at the request of psychiatrists and psychologists. Such occupational therapy was seen as an extension of psychodynamic approaches championed by other professionals rather than as a unique service. Indeed, several of the therapists in this survey spontaneously

---

*Barris, R. Toward an image of one's own: Sources of variation in the occupational therapist's role. Unpublished doctoral dissertation, Teachers College, Columbia University, 1983.

volunteered their feelings of insecurity regarding knowledge or the use of theory in psychosocial occupational therapy. Without a strong identity, they were lost in the pattern of ideas and actions represented in the psychosocial arena.

Chapter One, beings with a discussion of the history and purpose of occupational therapy knowledge. Chapter Two, examines how occupational therapy explains the well working or psychosocial health of humans. Chapter Three, discusses disorder, or how the occupational therapy body of knowledge views psychosocial problems. How a body of knowledge defines a problem or disorder determines how it will attempt resolution. This is the topic of the next chapter, action implications. Here, treatment prescribed by the occupational therapy body of knowledge is identified.

Two final chapters provide a perspective for critical evaluation. The criticisms and limitations chapter presents and interprets claims that have been made in the literature pertaining to the weaknesses or limitations of the occupational therapy body of knowledge. The final chapter reflects on the approach taken in this book.

What is identified as the unique occupational therapy contribution to the psychosocial arena reflects the authors' convictions about the unique orientation of occupational therapy in general. Thus, it should not be construed that the occupational therapy ideas forwarded in this text are essentially different from the approach that should be taken by occupational therapists in other areas of practice. It is the patient population which leads to differences in practice in the areas of physical and psychosocial dysfunction, not a difference in the body of knowledge that defines the roles and functions of occupational therapy.

The choice of certain words always presents a dilemma for writers; some of our choices bear mentioning. Every effort was made to eliminate sexist terminology throughout this volume. The terms "patients" and "clients" are both used throughout the text. Their use often reflects the context or setting being discussed. Thus, the term *client* was used in discussions of nontraditional situations, especially community mental health. *Patient* was used in discussions of more traditional medical circumstances. In addition, we used the term most often associated with the body of knowledge under discussion.

The term *psychosocial dysfunction* is used throughout the volume to refer to persons with (a) identified emotional disturbances, (b) mental retardation, and (c) developmental disabilities or physical problems that have precipitated a psychological or social disturbance. In reality these categories overlap. All have in common a disturbance to psychological and interpersonal well-being. More specific terms such as mental retardation,

OCCUPATIONAL THERAPY IN PSYCHOSOCIAL PRACTICE

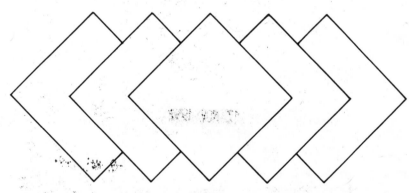

Roann Barris
Gary Kielhofner
Janet Hawkins Watts

SLACK Incorporated, 6900 Grove Road, Thorofare, New Jersey 08086

SLACK International Book Distributors

In Europe, the Middle East and Africa.
John Wiley & Sons Limited
Baffins Lane
Chichester, West Sussex P019 1UD
England

In Canada:
McAinsh and Company
2760 Old Leslie Street
Willowdale, Ontario M2K 2X5

In Australia and New Zealand:
MacLennan & Petty Pty Limited
P.O. Box 425
Artarmon, N.S.W. 2064
Australia

In Japan:
Central Foreign Books Limited
1-13 Jimbocho-Kanda
Tokyo, Japan

In Asia and India:
PG Publishing Pte Limited.
36 West Coast Road, #02-02
Singapore 0512

Foreign Translation Agent:
John Scott & Company
International Publishers' Agency
417-A Pickering Road
Phoenixville, PA 19460

Publisher: Harry C. Benson
Managing Editor: Lynn Borders
Editor: Stephanie Scanlon
Designer: Susan Hermansen
Production Coordinator: David Murphy

1574/12293

Printed in the United States of America

Library of Congress Catalog Card Number: 88-42960

ISBN: 1-55642-072-2

Published by: SLACK Incorporated
              6900 Grove Rd.
              Thorofare, NJ 08086

Last digit is print number: 10   9   8   7   6   5   4   3   2 schizophrenia, and the like were used when a particular topic pertained only to that subgroup of those with psychosocial dysfunction. Finally, we sought to avoid such terms as "mental retardates" and "the mentally ill," since such language does not acknowledge the human identity of these persons.

A glossary and summary table are provided as review and study guides. Reference lists provide additional readings for the interested person. We did attempt to provide complete excursion of relevant occupational therapy references.

Table of Contents

Occupational Therapy in Psychosocial Practice

1

The History and Purpose of Occupational Therapy

Although the field of occupational therapy formally came into existence only three-quarters of a century ago, the use of occupation as a form of treatment has a long and colorful history dating from the mid-eighteenth century. Quite remarkably, some fundamental concepts that emerged at that time have been preserved in occupational therapy and still constitute the core of its relevance and efficacy for those with psychosocial dysfunction. This is not to suggest that there has been a smooth progression of ideas and techniques over the past three centuries. On the contrary, the use of occupation as therapy for psychosocial problems died for a period of time and was reborn in this century.

Historical shifts and changes in psychosocial occupational therapy have been chronicled elsewhere.[2,3,9,14] The present purpose is to illuminate and order those central themes and practices that have endured. The underlying assumption is that those perennial elements that have survived are the core elements of psychosocial occupational therapy. Thus, this and the following chapters are not only descriptive but also prescriptive. That is, they offer a picture of how occupational therapy practice developed, and they propose a way of viewing and enacting occupational therapy in psychosocial practice.

The ideas and techniques that today are referred to as occupational therapy were stimulated in the past by concerns with the limitations of predominant methods of treatment. The earliest form of occupational therapy, referred to as moral treatment, emerged in the mid-eighteenth century as an alternative to the predominant abusive and punitive methods of responding to the insane. This moral treatment movement eventually died out. It was replaced with a medical model approach, which viewed mental illness as largely incurable and resulted in a custodial system of care. Modern occupational therapy emerged from the impetus of a few enlightened physicians and others as an alternative to the pessimism and inaction of the medical model.

MORAL TREATMENT: THE FIRST OCCUPATIONAL THERAPY

During the Middle Ages, persons with psychosocial dysfunction were largely neglected and abused. By the eighteenth century, it was common to incarcerate the mentally ill along with other problematic and indigent people. The dominant ideology of treatment was that the mentally ill needed to be imbued with fear. Thus, they were often frightened and tortured, albeit with therapeutic intentions.[10]

In reaction to these deplorable conditions, a number of reformers set out to turn the insane asylum into a place of genuine care. Moral treatment became the name for their movement. Moral treatment included not only the belief that patients needed kind and compassionate care but also the assertion that they should be engaged in the normal occupations of everyday life.

Moral treatment flourished because it worked, but also because the political and ideological climates of Western culture supported it. There was a growing optimism at the time that science would provide new answers and new hope for humanistic goals. The lawfulness of human behavior was stressed with a concomitant assertion that it could be systematically influenced. This led to the belief that those with psychosocial problems could be helped.[11] The optimistic belief that people had the potential for normal behavior also included the idea that some element of "normality" always remained within the person and that this remaining healthy aspect could be nurtured through moral treatment. In fact, the assumption that those with psychosocial problems possessed some degree of control and awareness was the basis for the proposal that they could be positively influenced by normal surroundings and routines of behavior.[1]

Bockoven[2] described moral treatment as an endeavor to awaken feelings of communality (a sense of belonging to a social group) in the mentally ill. This could be achieved through occupations "which required the patient to invest interest in something outside himself in cooperation with others, namely manual work, intellectual work, recreation, and religious worship" (pp. 75–76).[2] Bockoven went on to describe moral treatment as:

> organized group-living in which the integration and continuity of work, play and social activities produce a meaningful total life experience in which growth of individual capacity to enjoy life has maximum opportunity. (p. 76)[2]

Moral treatment was more than a reform and a method; it was also a philosophy of human nature and a theory of mental disorder that provided

2

a rationale for treatment. Bockoven's discussion of the fourfold meaning of the term "moral" is especially instructive for understanding what have always been the main themes of occupational therapy.[2] One meaning was close to what is meant by "morale," and it implied such emotions as enthusiasm, hope, confidence, and related feelings of well-being. Thinking about emotional disturbance, on the other hand, implied the opposite feelings of despair, lethargy, ennui, helplessness, and the like.

"Moral" also referred to mores or folkways, the ethos of normal conduct, and the meanings attached to a way of living. Thus, it connoted the confident and enthusiastic embracing of some recognizable external order (i.e., some cultural way of life) that had meaning for the person and resulted in a sense of well-being.

The third connotation was that the mentally ill were not responsible for their problems or culpable for their undesirable actions. This was an important step away from earlier interpretations that construed mental illness as moral degeneration and demonic possession. The fourth meaning was that society had an ethical obligation to care for less fortunate individuals.

One of the most interesting aspects of moral treatment is its view of the human mind and emotions. It was believed that all human thought was organized by the same underlying laws.[2] Thus, there was commonality in the human experience. In addition, the mind and the brain were seen as highly malleable and greatly influenced by physical and social surroundings.[11] The thrust of the occupations that filled the days of mental patients in moral treatment was to bring their thoughts and emotions into congruence with those of the larger community. This was to be accomplished not by force but by the gentle persuasion of participation in the occupations of a community.

In addition, there was also a perspective on how the mind worked and could be influenced by occupation. Licht quotes a discussion by Jarvis, a moral treatment writer:

As no two particles of matter can occupy the same point in space at the same moment, so no two absorbing thoughts or emotions can occupy the mind or heart at the same instant of time. So long then, as those, whose minds are prone to wander in delusions, are engaged in mechanical or other employments, their thoughts must be given exclusively to the conduct and succession of natural events and real processes; and as the mind can not admit or be possessed by both the sane and the insane idea, the insane one must be excluded, and the sane one reign paramount; all the mental powers of the worker which are in action for the moment are sane, and the mental disorder is for the moment, or that succession of moments, suspended. The sanity may be, and probably is, in most cases, broken and interrupted by insane thoughts and emotions. The attention to work may be, and undoubtedly often is, uncertain and fitful, and interspersed with sudden temporary alternations of order and disorder. The man may look at and think of his shoe, his awl and his hammer, and bring them together for a second, and let his crazed imagination carry his thoughts away into his delusions, or permit his morbid feeling to take possession of his soul, and absorb him in grief, or hate, or passion, or exuberant joy—but during that time, however short or long it may be, in which he is applying his awl to the leather, and lifting the hammer and striking the blow in the right place and with the intended effect, his mind must be given to the observation of those processes to see that they are conducted according to his plan; and, of course, his thought is sane, his hands are perfoming a sane act, the cerebral as well as the muscular movements are of the same character, and so much sanity is thereby developed and manifested. (pp. 11–12)[10]

This eloquent passage sums up the fundamental assertion of moral treatment that occupation brings the person into the order of the external world, which becomes imprinted on the mind and body.

The Demise of Moral Treatment

A number of interrelated changes in science, society, and medicine contributed to the decline of moral treatment. By the middle of the nineteenth century, American attitudes were rapidly changing. A massive influx of immigrants, many of whom were poor and indigent, resulted in growing prejudice, and asylums became overcrowded with what came to be known as the "insane foreign pauper."[2] With the emergence of Social Darwinism, the belief in a survival-of-the-fittest social dynamic and the concomitant conviction that people are not equal, the notion of a moral obligation for the care of the insane made less and less sense.

Science was also rapidly changing. In the previous era, scientific and humanistic goals had been united.[11] Science was now pursued for its own sake, and human problems often had to conform to its views and methods. Medicine's view of mental illness changed accordingly. Causes of mental illness were no longer ascribed to environmental pressures; rather, the new scientific perspective was that insanity was a disease with identifiable symptoms and a discoverable neurological cause.[11] Discovery of brain lesions in some patients gave impetus to the argument that mental illness was caused by brain disease. Because no cure for the faulty brain was known, this perspective led to growing pessimism about the curability of insanity.[2]

The crowding of hospitals and the economic concerns they posed also constrained the practice of moral treatment, which required an optimal ratio of patients to staff and pleasant surroundings. With growing pessimism about curability, it seemed unnecessary to allocate funds for the "superfluous" methods of moral treatment. Large asylums simply became warehouses for the hopelessly incurable. These alterations in social values, in economics, and in the population, combined with internal changes in medicine, led to a demise of moral treatment, and a period of custodialism ensued.

THE EMERGENCE OF OCCUPATIONAL THERAPY: A SECOND MORAL TREATMENT

In the first decades of this century, a number of persons reestablished moral treatment principles and techniques, labeling them occupational therapy. Several factors appear to have been instrumental in this reemergence. The study of psychological phenomena reawakened interest in emotional and cognitive factors in psychosocial problems, and the mental hygiene movement precipitated reforms in custodial care.[16] The most instrumental factor was the discontent of several physicians with the dominant medical model approach to psychiatry. Such physicians as Herbert Hall,[7] William Rush Dunton,[4] and Adolph Meyer[12] sought an alternate approach to the problems of mental illness. Their enthusiasm for and their theoretical and practical support of the occupational therapy movement was essential to its growth. In addition, a number of other leaders of varied backgrounds contributed to the early development of occupational therapy in psychosocial practice. Susan Tracy,[17] Louis Haas,[6] Eleanor Clarke Slagle,[15,16] Thomas Kidner,[8] and others represented such diverse interests and backgrounds as nursing, architecture, industrial arts, and social welfare.

The Thought of Early Occupational Therapy

Early occupational therapy was organized around the premise that human beings were complex creatures who required occupation in order to maintain their health:

> The whole of the human organization has its shape in a kind of rhythm. It is not enough that our hearts should be in a useful rhythm, always kept up to a standard at which it can meet rest as well as wholesome *strain* without upset. There are many other rhythms which we must be attuned to: the *larger* rhythms of night and day, of sleep and waking hours, of hunger and its gratification, and finally the big four—work and play and rest and sleep, which our organism must be able to balance even under difficulty. The only way to attain this balance in this is *actual doing, actual practice*, a program of wholesome living as the *basis* of wholesome feeling and thinking and fancy and interests. (p. 6)[12]

This statement embodies several fundamental tenets. First, human organisms are complex, and their organization is represented as a balance or rhythm. Second, that organization is dependent on the organism's occupation. Last, healthy mental states are the result of healthy occupational life-styles, and,

5

by implication, disturbed mental states can result from a breakdown of occupational life. Conversely, because of the importance of occupation in human life, it could be used to remediate loss of health:

> The development of the human brain is the result of man's struggle with the forces of nature throughout countless centuries and a continuous effort to adapt himself to his environment and provide for his own needs. Therefore, no more wholesome condition can be chosen for man than an environment of work, which when properly prescribed and controlled, can be of great value in restoring health. (p. 15)[6]

An Alternative View of Mental Illness

Early occupational therapists for the most part did not view mental illness through the medical model. Rather, they embraced a view of mental illness articulated by Adolph Meyer, in which habits, modes of adjustment, and environments were major factors.[13] Meyer's perspective came from many years of research with mentally ill patients. He discovered that the universal feature of their problems was a disorganization of habit.[2] He decried the medical model view that mental illness was a disease caused by some organic entity, and noted that "many formidable diseases are largely problems of adaptation and not some mysterious devil in disguise to be exorcised" (p. 1).[12] Meyer's theme of habit deterioration was echoed by Slagle, who noted that mental illness was largely a process of disorganized habits learned from exposure to disruptive environments.[15,16]

Dunton[4] and Kidner[8] emphasized the importance of habits balancing work, play, rest, and sleep and noted that a lack of leisure interests and pursuits, fatigue from overwork, exposure to monotonous and disinteresting work, and idleness could be sources of psychosocial problems.

Mental illness was viewed as a breakdown not only of patterns of behavior but also of the patterns of healthy emotion. This was generally expressed as a disruption of morale or demoralization. Those with mental problems were recognized as having lost interest, confidence, and hope, becoming isolated from their communities—all components of the process of demoralization.

The Rationale and Role of Occupation as a Remediative Measure

Quite naturally, the overall approach to remediation in early occupational therapy was to expose patients to tasks and pastimes in the context of normal daily and weekly routines. Dunton[4] was instrumental in developing much of the rationale for the mechanism of recovery or improvement from psychosocial problems through occupation. In his view, an important part of occupation for those with psychosocial problems was simply to maintain functional capacity and to prevent depression and other problems that result from inactivity.

A second important role of occupation was to correct faulty patterns of attention and behavior; activity acted as an antidote, drawing the patient into a state of mind and action opposite to the problematic one toward which he or she had a tendency. The following passage illustrates such an approach:

> In a case of dementia praecox where the subject is given to daydreaming or so-called mental rumination, occupation is given to keep the patient's train of thought in more healthy channels. In a case of mild excitement occupation will keep the patient's mind more continuously on one subject than is possible if he has not this stimulus to control his attention. (p. 25)[4]

A third aspect of occupation's influence on those with psychosocial problems was termed "substitution." It was generally accepted that mental illness involved the fusion of morbid and obsessive thoughts into the train of everyday consciousness. Occupation served as a means of replacing such thoughts with healthier ones generated in the course of interesting pastimes and tasks. This rationale was based on a continuation of the moral treatment idea that the mind could be occupied with only one dominant thought. Continued application to life tasks and interesting activities would eventually train the mind in patterns of healthy thought.

A fourth role of therapy was habit training.[15] Since people with psychosocial problems suffered from disorganized habit patterns, therapy would have to retrain them into adaptive patterns of living. Habits were thought to be acquired through practice and shaped by the social, temporal, and physical surroundings. Thus, patients would learn a healthy pattern of living only if they were exposed to a normal timetable of work, rest, play, and sleep; if they engaged in communal and cooperative tasks; and if they lived in pleasant surroundings that provided stimulation and opportunities for a variety of pursuits.[4,12,15]

A fifth aspect of occupational therapy was the restoration of morale, a social-psychological phenomenon.[4,16] Morale was the person's enthusiasm for a way of life. It was maintained through participation in a community's everyday life tasks and events. That is, morale was a feeling of interest, commitment, hope, and well-being supported by cultural and social meaning. It was thus reasoned that by exposing patients to meaningful pursuits of the culture, their morale could be restored.

Principles of Treatment

The roles of therapy implied several principles of treatment. The first principle found consistently in descriptions of occupational therapy was that it must arouse interest, courage, and confidence.[4,6,15,17] Methods of accomplishing this were the introduction of novel occupations that aroused curiosity, the personal interest of the therapist in the activity, the skillful presentation of activities to create arousal, and careful matching of the occupation to the patient's capacities and needs. This required the availability of a wide range of opportunities for action.

A second principle was that occupations should be applied with system and with precision.[4,8,16] This meant that the therapist had to pay careful attention to mental and physical limitations and abilities and to dispositions of the patient in order to choose and apply the proper occupations.[5] Similarly, consideration had to be given to the nature of the patient's problems and to the carefully planned presentation of occupations to counteract these problems.

A third treatment principle was that of gradation of occupations according to the increasing capacity of patients. Slagle articulates this principle as "grading the occupation from simple to complex, passing from the known to the unknown, increasing interest and requiring an increasing degree of concentration" (p. 15).[15] Gradation could be accomplished by varying a single activity or it might be embodied in a total program in which patients moved through phases of therapy.[6] For the most regressed patients in early occupational therapy, the first phase, habit training, was used to restore the basic skills and habits of self-care, giving the patient some degree of control over his or her immediate surroundings and over attention and action.[15] After habit training, patients progressed to work in an occupational therapy shop, which allowed them greater freedom to act and use skills.[8] The final phase of treatment was the pre-industrial or industrial therapy stage. Here patients worked in various industries of the hospital or in cottage industries maintained by the hospital under the supervision of lay workers. Occupational therapists served as consultants to those who supervised the patients in these work experiences. This progression from ward life to hospital industry helped assure the smooth transition of the patient from hospital to community life. It graded demands for performance so that the patient was gradually reorganized and gained increasing capacity, resulting in the ability to return to a more normal life.

A fourth principle was that occupational therapy focused on the health of patients rather than pathology and that it emphasized the expression of healthy emotions and attitudes.[4,6,16] This meant that occupation was not seen as a prescribed "remedy" but as something to be:

> followed for its own sake, . . . so that instead of being a medicine that can be dropped when the patient is cured, it has become rather a part of the restored individual's life, to be retained in some form as long as health exists. (p. 2)[5]

In order for occupational therapy to accomplish this goal, the ethos of the clinic had to differ from that of the ward and other therapies, where focus on pathology was more likely. One way of accomplishing this was that:

> A rigid rule against the discussion of symptoms or any matters relating to illness or treatment was enforced and the room became at once a cheery and attractive place. The atmosphere of interested activity prevailed. The work became the source of new purposes, of changed avenues of thought and of stimulated ambitions. . . . The evils of the idle association of nervous invalids were in a measure remedied, and a more positively wholesome spirit pervaded the institution. (p. 7.)[5]

In addition, the importance of having an esprit de corps, an atmosphere of cheerfulness, hope, industriousness, and order, was deemed critical. Haas[6] was especially articulate in this regard. He specified the details of both a physical plant and a social atmosphere that would positively influence patients. Haas,[6] Dunton,[4] and Hall[7] also stressed the importance of qualities such as craftsmanship and sportsmanship in the therapist and in the therapeutic occupations. If the occupations did not embody these wholesome and uplifting characteristics, they would not be therapeutic. Similarly, the therapist had to be patient, cheerful, enthusiastic, and resourceful in solving problems.[15,17]

A fifth principle was that occupational therapy had to be a total program of care. One of the most important facets of treatment in early occupational therapy was the recognition that it could not be limited to a few short sessions a week. Because most humans live in a balance of daily life occupations, total programs involving the activities of the patient's entire day were necessary for adequate treatment. It was further reasoned that without proper exposure to a total physical, social, and temporal environment the effects of occupational therapy on the patient would not be substantial. In order to effect such comprehensive programs, occupational therapists often had to assume roles as supervisors, consultants, and planners working with other disciplines and with laymen in the institution.

The knowledge and technology of early occupational therapy psychosocial practice appears more sophisticated than one would expect of a fledgling profession. However, if one considers that early occupational therapy was an extension of moral treatment—a long-standing approach to mental health— then it is not surprising that the field possessed a well-formulated tradition of knowledge. Despite its apparent coherence and viability, the early occupational therapy perspective came to be questioned deeply during the middle of this century. Eventually, it was largely dropped in favor of a more psychodynamically based version of occupational therapy.[9] When this happened, the view of mental illness, the rationale and role of occupations in therapy, and the principles of treatment changed in large measure. Psychoanalytic concepts promoted by psychiatrists as the most sophisticated and acceptable view of mental illness became the new conceptual foundation of psychosocial occupational therapy. Thus, humans were viewed primarily as tension-reducing organisms driven by unconscious forces. Problems of mental illness were seen as anxiety states and failures of ego maturation. Therapy focused on the expression of feelings through activity and the gratification of primitive needs. Occupation was no longer viewed as an important force in maintaining the organization of human behavior, but rather as one of several vehicles (talk being the predominant one) through which patients could therapeutically fulfill needs and express feelings. Some therapists came to see occupations as only secondary to the process of establishing a verbal relationship with clients, and eventually some therapists abandoned occupation altogether in favor of purely verbal methods of treatment.

Occupational therapists soon recognized that this shift in psychosocial practice had taken the field away from its original purpose, knowledge, and practice. This resulted in a new series of efforts to articulate and shape theory and practice in a manner consistent with the moral treatment and early occupational therapy traditions. Thus, modern occupational therapy in psychosocial practice is once again returning to its core concepts and practice. The remaining chapters illustrate the elements of theory and practice that reflect this continuity.

SUMMARY

Moral Treatment

The history of using occupation as therapy began with the moral treatment movement of the mid-18th to mid-19th centuries.

Moral treatment was a humanistic treatment of mentally ill persons that stressed compassion and the commonality of the human condition.

Moral treatment was based on the scientific view that human behavior was subject to certain discoverable laws and that the environment influenced the mind and body. Thus, the possibility of remediating problems of mental illness was viewed with optimism.

Moral treatment had four connotations:

1. morale, or the enthusiasm, hope, confidence, and well-being that supported and resulted from involvement in one's everyday world;
2. the ethos of normal conduct—that is, mores or folkways reflecting the order and meanings of the culture;

3. the lack of culpability of mentally ill persons for their actions and their right to compassion; and
4. society's moral obligation to care for the mentally ill.

Occupation was used in moral treatment to bring persons into interaction with their environments so that the order of the external world was imprinted on the mind and body.

Moral treatment subsided despite its empirical success because of changes in science, medicine, and social values.

Early Occupational Therapy

Early occupational therapy was a reemergence of moral treatment ideas and practices.

The thought of early occupational therapy stressed that:
1. humans were complex beings whose bodies and minds were organized into a balance or rhythm;
2. occupation (i.e., doing the tasks of daily life provided by one's culture) was necessary to maintain the organization and balance of humans; and
3. the organization of behavior is reflected in human habits.

Early occupational therapy viewed mental illness as:
1. a reaction to the environment and a disorganization of rhythm and balance instead of a disease caused by some germ or trauma;
2. a manifestation of disrupted or maladaptive habits; and
3. a form of demoralization that resulted from poor occupational life-styles or disruption of occupation.

The rationale and role of occupation as a remediative measure was:
1. to maintain functional capacity and prevent depression and other problems that resulted from inactivity;
2. to correct faulty patterns of attention and behavior;
3. to substitute healthy thoughts for pathological thoughts by orienting the patient to life tasks;
4. to train persons in correct habits of behavior needed for competence; and
5. to restore morale for living.

Principles of treatment were:
1. that occupation should arouse interest, courage, and confidence through the qualities of the occupation and the therapist's skill and interest in the occupation;
2. that occupation must be applied with precision to match the strengths and weaknesses and the personal dispositions of the patient;

11

3. that occupation should be graded from simple to complex to provide a continuum of reorganization of behavior;
4. that therapy should focus on health rather than pathology and that the clinic should reflect concern with the normal life of the culture; and
5. that occupational therapy was a total program of care that organized the patient's entire daily activity.

Early occupational therapy was drastically changed because of pressure from medicine, and it became largely a psychoanalytic treatment for a period of time.

Current efforts seek to return occupational therapy to its traditional role and practices

REFERENCES

1. Bing, R. Occupational therapy revisited: A paraphrasic journey. *American Journal of Occupational Therapy*, 1981, *35*, 499–518.
2. Bockoven, J. S. *Moral treatment in community mental health*. New York: Springer, 1972.
3. Diasio, K. Psychiatric occupational therapy: Search for a conceptual framework in light of psychoanalytic ego psychology and learning theory. *American Journal of Occupational Therapy*, 1968, *22*, 400–414.
4. Dunton, W. R. *Occupational therapy: A manual for nurses*. Philadelphia: W. B. Saunders, 1915.
5. Fuller, D. The need of instruction for nurses in occupations for the sick. In S. Tracy (Ed.), *Studies in invalid occupation*. Boston: Whitcomb & Barrows, 1912.
6. Haas, L. *Practical occupational therapy*. Milwaukee: Bruce Publishing Co., 1944.
7. Hall, H. *Occupational therapy: A new profession*. Concord: Rumford Press, 1923.
8. Kidner, T. B. *Occupational therapy: The science of prescribed work for invalids*. Stuttgart: W. Kohlhammer, 1930.
9. Kielhofner, G., & Burke, J. P. The evolution of knowledge and practice in occupational therapy: Past, present and future. In G. Kielhofner (Ed.), *Health through occupation: Theory and practice in occupational therapy*. Philadelphia: F. A. Davis, 1983.
10. Licht, S. *Occupational therapy sourcebook*. Baltimore: Williams & Wilkins, 1948.
11. Magaro, P., Gripp, R., & McDowell, D. *The mental health industry: A cultural phenomenon*. New York: John Wiley & Sons, 1978.

12. Meyer, A. The philosophy of occupational therapy. *Archives of Occupational Therapy*, 1922, *1*, 1–10.
13. Mora, G. Theories of personality and psychopathology: III. Other psychoanalytic and related schools. Adolph Meyer. In Freedman, Kaplan, & Sadock (Eds.), *Comprehensive textbook of psychiatry II* (Vol. 1) (2nd ed.). Baltimore: Williams & Wilkins, 1975.
14. Mosey, A. C. Involvement in the rehabilitation movement—1942–1960. *American Journal of Occupational Therapy*, 1971, *25*, 234–236.
15. Slagle, E. C. Training aides for mental patients. *Archives of Occupational Therapy*, 1922, *1*, 11–17.
16. Slagle, E. C., & Robeson, H. *Syllabus for training of nurses in occupational therapy* (2nd ed.). Utica, N.Y.: State Hospitals Press, 1941.
17. Tracy, S. *Studies in invalid occupation.* Boston: Whitcomb & Barrows, 1912.

2

The View of Order in Occupational Therapy

✳Order is viewed in occupational therapy as the individual's ability to competently perform the everyday tasks✳and behaviors✳of life and to gain satisfaction from this performance.[25,43] Work, play, and self-care have been identified as the major areas of daily life performance. Collectively they are referred to as occupational behavior[32] or occupational performance.[48] Thus, the view of order in occupational therapy can be described as focusing on people's ability for occupational behavior or performance.

In occupational therapy, a person can be recognized as having a disease process (e.g., Down's syndrome) and still exhibit order, since the capacity for occupational behavior can exist concurrently with certain diseases. Similarly, people may simultaneously exhibit some pathological symptoms (e.g., hallucinations or anxiety) and still be able to function adequately and, thus, be considered in a state of order. Conversely, occupational therapists do not assume that because a pathological state or symptom is removed that order automatically follows. There is a tendency in psychiatry to assume that once a patient's symptoms are allayed with medication or when anxiety is reduced through verbal therapy, that competence will be a natural sequel. This is not the case. Order is a state of organization for productive and playful functioning that requires the integrity and interrelationship of many components of the human being.

Several major themes generated in occupational therapy to explain and describe order can be delineated: (1) humans as open systems, (2) intrinsic motivation, (3) humans as decision makers, (4) roles as organizers of behavior, (5) temporal adaptation, (6) person-environment interaction, and (7) occupational performance components.

In this chapter, we will examine each of these themes and the ways in which they illuminate order in human occupational behavior. These themes overlap and collectively constitute an overall view of order.

HUMAN BEINGS AS OPEN SYSTEMS

Open system concepts represent an interdisciplinary movement in the sciences aimed at generating a more adequate conceptualization of living phenomena.[5,50] Open systems concepts attempt to go beyond thinking of living systems as machine-like, to acknowledge that they are more complex than inanimate, closed systems. Open system concepts have been identified by several occupational therapy writers as being relevant to explaining order in the occupational behavior of humans.[10,13,16,20,25,39,52] This section provides an overview of systems concepts and how they are being used to conceptualize order in occupational therapy.

Self-Maintaining Systems

The fundamental property of the open system is the capacity for self-maintenance and self-change through the system's own action. An open system, to use the Fidlers' phrase, can become through doing.[13] This property is present in all living systems.

The way in which an open system maintains and changes itself through doing or action is explained by the concept of a cycle. In the open system, the cycle is a self-repeating process, involving four interrelated stages.[20,25] *Intake** is the importation of energy and information from the environment. *Throughput* is the transformation of the energy or information into some other form and its incorporation into the system's structure and process. In the throughput phase, the system often changes itself to accommodate incoming information. *Output* is the behavior or action of the system. In the final stage, *feedback*, information concerning the progress and consequences of action (output), is returned to the system. It then becomes part of the intake of the system. As this feedback enters the system, it is used in the throughput stage to adjust and rearrange internal components.

This cycle is an ongoing process. The system takes in information, transforms the information and itself, acts, generates feedback, incorporates it, and so on. Because of the nature of this cycle, the open system's action (output) is critical for maintaining and changing its structures. Open system processes permeate all of human existence and behavior. The act of reading this book is a process of taking in information; interpreting it and incorporating it into

---

*Intake is used here instead of the more common term *input*. The change is to reflect the active nature of intake. People do not passively receive information from their environments; they seek out and selectively take in information.

16

one's understanding and memory (throughput); eventually using it in some fashion, such as responding to an exam or designing patient treatment (output); and thus generating consequences that can be used to evaluate the knowledge and how well one has incorporated and used it (feedback). The outcome of one's use of the information (in an exam or in the clinic) will shape further action and decisions for action. Thus, what one does will further influence what one becomes and what one will do in the future.

The importance of the open cycle for maintaining and changing the system can further be appreciated from the perspective of another property of open systems, the primacy of function over structure. Closed systems (i.e., inanimate systems such as machines) function only in ways determined by their structure. For instance, a car engine's functions are totally specified by the internal structure of its parts. In an open system, the relationship is somewhat reversed. Rather than function being totally dependent on structure, structure largely depends on function. Process or function is basic to the open system. Structure is always changing and results from processes underlying the open system. This becomes more apparent if we consider an example such as the development of a human being. The structure of the human from the stage of the fertilized ovum through adulthood is constantly changing. That structure is first determined by the functions of cell division and a plethora of other physiological events that occur in sequence with intricate interrelationships. Later, especially from the period of birth, the function of the human being becomes a determinant of evolving structures in the musculoskeletal, nervous, and personality systems. The action of the child facilitates nervous pathways, increases muscle strength and bone mass, and develops cognitive and perceptual abilities. These are a few of the many facets of the system that must be developed through the system's action.

Particularly relevant to psychosocial practice is the open system concept that a person's life experiences (the ongoing cycles of output, feedback, intake, and throughput) shape and determine abilities, preferences, self-assessment, values, and other variables critical to psychosocial adaptation. This concept parallels the Fidlers' discussion of doing:

> *Doing* is viewed as enabling the development and integration of sensory, motor, cognitive, and psychosocial systems; serving as a socializing agent; and verifying one's efficacy as a competent, contributing member of one's society. (p. 305)[13]

Thus, to say that a human being is an open system is to say that what he or she is and becomes is a function of what he or she does. This not only provides a foundation for understanding order in the human system, but it also spells the basic rationale underlying the therapeutic approach of occupational therapy. Engaging people in purposeful tasks, play, and other occupations is a means of shaping their doing (output) and thereby influencing change. This change may be in the nervous system, in the person's beliefs about self, in the ability to perform some skill, or in a variety of other dimensions.

Hierarchy

Another system concept that is critical to the view of order is hierarchy. In an open system, hierarchy refers to the way in which parts are organized into a gestalt, or meaningful whole.[20,41] The functional components of a system are arranged in different levels with specific relationships between the levels.[22] Higher levels in a hierarchy govern lower levels. Lower levels constrain higher levels; that is, by virtue of their own abilities and limitations, they set limits on what higher levels can command them to do.

We can observe a hierarchy in the functional aspects of the human body. At the lowest level is the musculoskeletal system. This system consists of the structures that enable movement. The next higher level is the nervous system, which commands and governs musculoskeletal action. In turn, the nervous system is constrained from commanding what the musculoskeletal system is not capable of performing.

In the psychosocial practice arena, an important aspect of the hierarchy of human function is the relationship of the musculoskeletal system to the nervous system, of the nervous system to the symbolic or conscious system, and of the latter to the social system. According to hierarchical principles, the nervous system, which governs the musculoskeletal system, is commanded and governed by human consciousness and in turn constrains that consciousness.[21,22,28,41] By the same token, the social system gives commands to the individual through norms and role expectations. The individual and his or her capabilities, in turn, constrain the social system's ability to command behavior. For example, a family may place a high value on academic performance, thus influencing a child's efforts in school. If, however, the child has limited intellectual capacity, the family's expectations for high academic achievement cannot be fulfilled. Levels of function and structure are thus intimately interrelated in the human open system.

Work and Play as Output

Work and play have been conceptualized as the output of the open system.[25] Play contributes to the development of competence. Early childhood play develops sensory motor abilities,[29,33] rules (or internal images) that guide competent action,[41,42] and understanding of various roles and their requirements.[26] Play is an effective learning medium because it is free of overwhelming consequences. In play, the individual has freedom of exploration and can express creative and risk-taking behaviors.[41,49]

In adolescence, play serves as an arena for further developing interactional skills and for socializing with one's peers.[2,41,45] The hobbies of adolescence allow expression of personal mastery. In adulthood, play generally serves as an antidote to work, providing relaxation and recommitting the individual to the realities and demands of the work world.[40] Adult play (especially in the form of such cultural rituals as the celebration of holidays) serves an important function of reaffirming the values of the culture and social group. For example, sports express the American values of competition, teamwork, and giving one's best.

Work is important to the individual as an arena for expressing interests and values and for developing self-esteem.[17,45] Since work is valued by the culture, those who work experience a sense of personal worth through their contribution to the social group. Work begins with childhood chores and self-care and progresses through the paid and unpaid productive tasks of adult life.

Occupational therapy has always recognized the importance of play and work for maintaining health. Open system concepts allow the field to conceptualize how occupation organizes and changes the system. As output, the occupational behaviors of play and work are important for the development of capacities and commitments in childhood and for their maintenance in adulthood. Both work and play must exist in order for the person to be healthy.[45] When robbed of access to these occupations, the basic cycle of the open system is interrupted and degeneration follows.

INTRINSIC MOTIVATION

Early occupational therapy was based on the conviction that humans needed to engage in occupations. The field sought to extend its original concept by incorporating emerging theories of motivation. The major concepts of motivation in the first half of this century were generated by adherents of behaviorism and psychoanalysis. These theories share a view of human beings as passive creatures seeking equilibrium through tension reduction. They also view humans as driven by forces over which they have little control. They are diametrically opposed, however, in that behaviorism considers behavior to be environmentally determined, while psychoanalysis sees it as being psychically or inner-determined. According to both these theories, occupation is not a direct motive or need of humans. Behaviorism resulted in the view that people engage in work and play because it was a means to satisfy drives and thereby was reinforced (e.g., working in order to be able to buy food). Psychoanalysis suggested that occupation was an activity that mediated un-

19

conscious drives through symbolism. For instance, hammering could be a way of acting out aggressive drives, or boring a hole in wood might have the symbolic meaning of releasing sexual tension.

While both theories offered plausible explanations for occupational behavior, they suggested that it was extrinsically motivated. That is, it was done not for its own sake but for some ulterior motive. For a period of time, occupational therapists sought to incorporate these theories into the field's view of human behavior and to develop related treatment approaches.

Eventually therapists began to view these theories as unsatisfactory because they offered no direct explanation of the motive for occupation.[11,14] These therapists pointed to new theories that offered better explanations. Theories of intrinsic motivation emerged from the efforts of behavioral scientists to include a drive for action, stimulation, competition, achievement, arousal, and like experiences. Intrinsic motivation theories shared the common themes that humans engaged in action for its own sake without the benefit of extrinsic reinforcement or unconscious motivation. In short, they recognized another major motive in human behavior that complemented and counterbalanced the motive of seeking equilibrium or tension reduction. This motive was one of tension-seeking, leading to change and growth in the organism.

Intrinsic motivation has been identified as the underlying dynamic of occupational behavior and the motivational force best suited to the occupational therapy clinic.[1,14] Recognizing intrinsic motivation as the basis of occupation allowed the field to speak of occupation as a basic human need. Further, it led to a greater understanding of the dynamics of occupation in human life.

Whereas psychoanalytic and behavioral thought show how extrinsic motives are useful to the organism's survival, intrinsic motivation theories point to another major function in human life. By seeking activity for its own sake, organisms encounter new events, objects, and people; generate new experiences for themselves; and, in the course of so doing, learn and change. Intrinsic motivation is thus recognized as the basic force underlying change and growth in the person. In terms of the open system, intrinsic motivation leads systems to produce output and thus energizes the basic cycle of the system, facilitating its maintenance and change.

Intrinsic motivation theory emphasizes the critical nature of childhood play for development. Children engage in play for its own sake.[14] The motive of play is a drive for exploration manifest in an attitude of curiosity in the child. Children develop competence when they curiously explore their environments; that is, through play and exploration they learn to act successfully in and on the human and nonhuman environment by rules of competent behavior.[41,42]

The intrinsic motive also maintains competence in adult life. The exploratory drive of childhood is translated into a drive for competence and later for achievement.[41] As individuals develop and acquire basic abilities, their need for stimulation leads to a search for greater challenge. Finding out how to manipulate the environment leads to being able to perform tasks with a degree of mastery, and finally to the ability to accomplish things according to standards of excellence or in comparison to the accomplishments of others. These motives underlie the productive contributions of people to society. The motive for early play becomes the motive for productive participation in the family and in a succession of social institutions throughout life.

In addition to generating skills that support competence, intrinsic motives also lead to behaviors that generate feelings of accomplishment, satisfaction, and effectiveness. Feelings of efficacy are critical to the ongoing competent behavior of people because they generate a sense of hopefulness.[47] The concept of personal causation elaborates this point.[26] Personal causation refers to the person's drive to be a cause, to have effects. People who are successful in their interactions with the environment develop a sense of personal causation, which leads them to confidently seek out opportunities for action and challenges for behavior.

Intrinsic motivation in the human system is not just a compelling force that drives humans; it is a process of choosing or willing one's course of action.[25] This volitional aspect of humans means that humans are decision makers. The decisions underlying the process of exploring and mastering one's world through occupation are a basic force in the dynamics of the human system and its maintenance of order.[25]

HUMANS AS DECISION MAKERS

A perennial theme in occupational therapy is the importance of personal control and self-determination. In concert with the theme of intrinsic motivation, which directed attention to people's internal and conscious reasons for engaging in occupation, several concepts have been developed which further delineate the dynamics of how and why people make choices about occupation. Included are the concepts of interests and values and the developmental process of occupational choice.

The decision to engage in particular occupations is informed by the meaning these activities have for an individual.[9] Occupations derive their meanings from the culture's view and definition of them and from an individual's values and personal interpretation of past and present experiences. In a culture, certain occupations may be highly central, imbued with the values of the group, and capable of signifying a range of emotions and convictions. For example, Thanksgiving dinner signifies values of family and country, freedom and plenty; it evokes emotions of well-being and gratitude, and it recommits people to these fundamental values. Other activities have meanings that are highly personal and determined from a lifetime of experience. Cynkin[9] points out, for instance, that the simple act of making a pie can signify personal competence, security, a sense of order and calm and productivity. The meanings of other occupations may be largely in their intrinsic pleasure, the satisfaction and interest they generate. Still other meanings of activities lie in their relationship to accomplishing goals. Completing an exam or a semester of courses is all the more significant when it means nearing the goal of completing a degree and entering a chosen profession. Occupational behavior is maintained when the person finds meaning in it. Meaning is thus an important dimension of order in human occupation.

Interests

Interests are affective phenomena that influence one's choices.[31] They are preferences for types of objects, people, or activities because of their ability to afford enjoyment.[4,21]

Matsutsuyu[31] elaborated the meaning of interests in six propositions: (a) interests are influenced by the family through socialization; (b) interests bring forth affective responses to objects, persons, and ideas; (c) interests determine choices for action; (d) interests are important to action that is personally satisfying; (e) interests can maintain persistent action; and (f) interests reflect a person's awareness of his or her areas of ability and identity. As these propositions illustrate, interests are important components of individuals' personalities that influence what action they will choose and why it is likely to be enjoyable.

Interests are important organizers of behavior because the internal priority of interests enables one to choose among alternatives for action and to establish a pattern of behavior for satisfying use of time.[25] Without interests, a person's ability to make consistent choices is obstructed and the individual is less disposed to interact with the environment.

Social approval and personal success influence what likes and dislikes a person will develop.[4] In addition, the development of interests is a function of the individual's participation in activity. The individual who lacks motivation and who fails to explore and experiment will tend to lack interests. Thus, whether people have well-defined interests depends on their initial opportunities to act on an innate tendency to explore and master the environment and receive feedback on various activities.

Values

Individuals possess a value orientation or collection of personal images of what is good, right, or important. This value orientation reflects a person's set of priorities for behavior; these priorities, in turn, guide the formation of operational goals, which influence choices for behavior.[25] Values vary among cultural subgroups[27] and include notions of time use, the importance of types of work, and achievement through competition versus cooperation. Values are intimately related to the meaningfulness of activities and to their significance for security and a sense of worth and importance.

Occupational behavior and, similarly, the collective societal understanding of what constitutes normal or abnormal behavior are culturally determined through the influence of society's value system.[27] For example, societal values, such as the "Protestant work ethic," have had a major impact in determining the way people view and use time.[19] These collectively acknowledged social values are acquired through childhood socialization, the child's observation of or instruction in what characteristic behavior is required by the larger culture. As individuals acknowledge the obligatory nature of values, they come to perceive them as compelling their own behavior.

Because people attach emotions to their values, they generally feel compelled to conform to these values or they experience a personal sense of failure or guilt. On the other hand, values are a source of positive emotion, because they carry the meaning of belonging to a social group and provide a sense of personal identity. When a person operationalizes values in occupational behavior, he or she experiences a feeling of doing the right thing, being a good or valuable person, and meeting social obligations. Thus, values both define and shape behavior.

Occupational Choice

The course of development toward adult life is punctuated by an important process of choosing one's life work.[22,39,52] Occupational choice begins in childhood and typically extends through late adolescence in this culture. Originally thought to be an irreversible process, it is now recognized as something people may do more than once as they make major occupational changes in adult life (e.g., changing a career or preparing for retirement).

The first period of occupational choice, which roughly corresponds to early childhood, is labeled the fantasy period. During this time, choices are not constrained by reality and they are ordinarily made solely on the basis of the perceived pleasure associated with the occupation. For instance, the child may choose to be Superman when he or she grows up because of the "fun" of being able to fly and having superhuman strength. The tentative period, which occurs during the second half of middle childhood and in early adolescence, is a time of making provisional choices based on a clearer assessment of personal interests, capacity, and value. These three considerations are delineated as stages within this period. First, choices are made primarily on the basis of likes or dislikes; then they are considered in terms of one's assessment of personal ability; and finally choices are considered on the basis of social values as the person seeks to have a place in the social group. A final stage in the tentative period is termed the transitional stage. This is when the adolescent begins to take steps toward enacting the choice (e.g., getting a degree or training).

The realistic period, which has three stages, is next. In the exploratory stage, the older adolescent takes a closer look at the chosen occupation and the opportunities it provides for satisfaction and security. During the next step, crystallization, alternative choices are more fully explored and the person narrows the choice down to a particular field. Finally, in the specification stage, the individual delineates any specialization within the chosen occupation. This stage often occurs during or just after the period of actual training for the occupation.

Occupational choice is a complex process by which individuals shape their commitment to a particular kind of work and invest both emotional energy and effort into identification with and preparation for a line of work. Occupational choice is an important determinant of the degree of stability and satisfaction a person is likely to experience in his or her career. This process is very much influenced by a person's successes and failures throughout development, consequent self-perceptions, opportunities to explore alternatives, and the presence of adult role models.[39]

Occupational choice is not altogether a process of free self-determination. The individual must seek to balance and optimize several factors. Economic, personal, and social factors may constrain one's ability to make a given choice. An occupation that maximizes one desirable factor may lack another. Ultimately, the choice reflects a series of compromises and reconsiderations that attempt to fit most of the requirements of the individual and the environment.

ROLE AS AN ORGANIZER OF BEHAVIOR

The concept of role was brought into occupational therapy from the social sciences because it provides a means of explaining much of people's regulated behavior.[7] A role is a "position in society that contains a set of expected responsibilities and privileges" (p. 226).[3] Roles have two components: an internal component, pertaining to how the person experiences and acts on his or her roles, and an external component, consisting of ascribed status and expectations for behavior. The role is at once a status and a set of obligations necessary for the maintenance of some social group. For example, the role of a homemaker has classically been an important position necessary for the maintenance of the family. Roles are also a source of identity and a guide for behavior to the people in the roles. They provide avenues through which people can achieve a sense of competence. Thus, the role helps match the needs of the person to the needs of the social group.

The Internalized Role

The concept of internalized role refers to roles that have been incorporated into one's behavior and self-perception.[25] These internalized roles serve as a frame of reference for people as they act in everyday life, defining what and how they should perform. For example, people generally consider themselves to be in a worker role from 9 a.m. to 5 p.m. during the work week. At other times, they may perceive themselves to be in parent, spouse, volunteer, or other roles. This does not mean that they consciously categorize all their behavior and think specifically of being in a role at any given time. However, subtle perceptions of being in a role do shape ongoing personal experience. For example, many people put on a uniform to signal to themselves and others that they are assuming the worker role. When one comes home from work, a change of clothes may again signal a role change. Behavior also changes as one leaves one role for another; the manner in which one speaks to a spouse, a co-worker, and a child varies quite predictably around the expectations and functions of the respective roles.

Each person has a unique and sometimes changing perception of the requirements of any role. Newly married people often learn that each has different expectations of what they should do as spouses. A new worker often finds that his or her perceptions of what is required on the job must change to accommodate predetermined job requirements. Some people expect more of themselves than others do in a given role; other people expect too little and, thereby, are deemed incompetent in the role. Still others may have inappropriate ideas of what is required of them, causing problems in the social system to which the role belongs. Internalized expectations are thus seen as important determinants of how well a person performs in a given role.

People ordinarily assume several roles at any point in their lives. A child is typically a player, a family member, and a student. An adult may be a worker, spouse, parent, volunteer, and hobbyist. A person must be able to balance these roles and their demands as well as the opportunities they provide for satisfying experiences. Balance includes being able to fit role performance comfortably into one's schedule, having sufficient variety in the types of role activities one performs, and having sufficient roles to fill one's time meaningfully.

Organizing Effects of Role

The organizing effects of role derive from the fact that one's set of roles prescribe time use, normative guides for behavior, and standards of competency. Everyday use of time is, for the most part, structured by a succession of roles.[3,19] For instance, a working woman may find that her succession of roles includes being homemaker, worker, and homemaker again at the end of the day. In daily life, one may often perform two roles simultaneously and may interrupt one role to perform some duty belonging to another role.

Roles also carry with them unique expectations for behavior and demeanor. For instance, work roles may include expectations for how one dresses and talks, what attitudes one exhibits, and how one relates to peers, supervisors, and subordinates. Each role has its own ambience. For instance, some roles require formal behavior while others allow more freedom. The ability to discriminate these fine points of role requirements is important for successful role performance.

Finally, each role has a set of built-in requirements that set minimum standards for competence. Often, these are formalized in job descriptions or made explicit in orientations and other verbal exchanges. At other times, they may be negotiated, as when spouses decide how to share household duties. Failure to live up to these basic demands of the role constitutes role incompetence and invariably evokes negative reactions from others in the social system.

In summary, the roles one possesses organize behavior by determining how time will be used, by influencing subtle demeanor and attitudes, and by specifying what performances are expected. The degree to which roles actually exert this organizing influence is determined by how clear expectations are made in the environment, how accurately the individual has internalized them, and the process of negotiation and compromise that occurs when internalized and external expectations do not match.[15]

Role Careers and Socialization

The course of occupational development has been described as the occupational career.[3] It involves a series of role shifts that is partly socially determined and partly a matter of personal choice. For example, in our society a typical succession of roles over the life span is player, student, worker, and retiree. People are expected to make a transition from one role to the next at fairly specific ages. In some cases, there are even laws to enforce these role transitions (e.g., mandatory education and retirement)

Heard conceptualizes the process of acquiring new roles as an open system process.[15] The intake to the system is the expectations that go with a given role. At this stage, the person negotiates between his or her own expectations for a role and those of the external society that is setting the priorities. The next phase, throughput, occurs when a person begins to sift through and select alternatives for role behavior that suit the role demands. Output is the actual role behavior that the person produces. Through feedback, the person learns about the success of his or her performance in meeting role demands. This results in adjustments in role behavior to better meet role demands.

Through socialization, individuals learn what roles they are expected to assume and what they should do in these roles.[3] Socialization begins with the play of children. During this time, they observe many adult roles and begin to try them out. For example, dramatic play (e.g., playing house) gives the child a chance to see what it might be like to perform adult roles. Later, children find out they are expected to enter school and therein learn a whole new set of demands for performance. Concurrently, children experience an increase in expectations for contributing to their own self-maintenance and to the maintenance of the household through chores. This gradual process prepares the young person for entry into the more demanding roles of adult life.

Socialization does not cease once one has reached adulthood.[15] Each time a person changes jobs, enters into a new role through marriage, joins a church or social group, or becomes a volunteer, there is a period of socialization during which the person learns the particular expectations and requirements of the new role.

Transitions from role to role require reorganization on the part of the individual and can be adaptively challenging.[19] Major role transitions (e.g., from student to worker or from worker to retiree) place demands on the individual to reorganize the use of time in daily life. Often, the individual will be required to learn new skills and to reorganize habits of daily life to find new sources of identity and satisfaction.[25] On the other hand, past role success is viewed as a resource for current role adaptation. The history of role performance tends to influence a person's success in roles.[34]

The Range of Occupational Roles

When role theory was incorporated into occupational therapy, three major classes of roles were identified: personal-sexual, familial, and occupational. The latter were noted as the primary concern of occupational therapy.[34]

It now appears more accurate to suggest that an individual role (e.g., a spouse) might have both personal-sexual and occupational aspects. A spouse must not only relate affectively and sexually to a partner, but also perform certain tasks related to maintaining a common household. To view roles in this way would appear to preserve the intention of earlier writers—that is, to focus on roles that demand performance in life tasks—while providing a more accurate and complete way of describing roles within which a person can engage in occupational behaviors. Following this rationale, Oakley[37] developed the following taxonomy of occupational roles: participant in an organization, hobbiest/amateur, friend, family member, care-giver, home maintainer, student, religious participant, worker, and volunteer.

TEMPORAL ADAPTATION

The theme of time or temporal adaptation is one of the earliest and most central concepts of occupational therapy. Today, occupation is still generally defined in occupational therapy as one's use of time in productive and playful pursuits.

A conceptual framework of temporal adaptation was formulated by Kielhofner[19] as a means of viewing how people ordered their daily and developmental behavior. For human beings, the awareness and experience of time is a reality so fundamental that it influences and directs all action. Temporal adaptation is defined as the organization of daily life behavior on an ongoing basis. Two aspects of human temporality are stressed—the internal image of time and the organization of time use.

Internal Image of Time

Human beings have an internal image of time, a temporal framework shaped by the prevalent culture and personal experiences. Each culture carries with it definitions of time, values concerning time, and prescriptions for the use of time. For instance, Americans tend to view time as a finite commodity that they can compartmentalize and thus schedule, save or waste, spend or sell. This view and valuation of time leads most Americans to feel an obligation to profitably fill time with activity. Further, persons may be judged incompetent when they habitually waste or cannot manage time.

Socialization exposes people to the temporal framework of their culture. If they successfully incorporate cultural attitudes and prescriptions concerning time use, they will be better able to meet the demands of their social environments. Time perspective is also an individual matter. Childhood and later experiences result in a set of individual attitudes about time and a collection of images or rules for how to organize and use time. These rules range from simple learnings about how to sequence behaviors in time, to complex time management practices needed in adult life. Time perspective also includes one's view of self in time. Culturally derived norms specify how a person should progress in his or her lifetime (e.g., from player to student to worker), when such transitions should take place, and how a person should behave at a given age. People generally see themselves as progressing along a time continuum and thereby plan for the future. Future orientation and goals organize present action by placing demands on and setting priorities for how one uses time.

Interrelated with one's temporal perspective are the values and interests that people use as a guide to making decisions. Barring environmental and other constraints, people's healthy use of time reflects the activities that they find interesting or valuable. Thus, it can be seen that the temporal perspective of an individual is a complex network of images that guide how a person plans, organizes, and uses time in everyday life and over the life span.

Organization of Time Use

The second aspect of temporality is the organization of time use. There is a natural order to daily life represented in a balance of work, play, and self-maintenance.[19] This balance consists not only of adequate amounts of each behavioral domain in daily life, but also on the interdependence of each. Work success requires performance of self-maintenance activities such as hygiene and dressing. Play serves to refresh and energize the individual for work. Play is earned through the work of adulthood. Consequently, these behaviors exist in a dynamic balance necessary for healthy existence.[44]

In order to achieve an organization of time that reflects this adaptive balance, a person must develop a routine. The regulator of temporal organization is habit. Kielhofner notes that "habits are instantaneous automatic choices of action made throughout the day . . . organizing temporal behavior to meet societal requirements for competence" (p. 239).[19] Habits serve to organize a person's skills into regular sequences and to order them in the context of the day and week.[24,25] Habits (along with roles) maintain the output or behavior of a person, organizing behavior so that it fulfills both the demands of the external environment and the internal needs of the individual.[24] This is illustrated through the simple routine of activities of daily living. Getting up in the morning, bathing, and dressing may meet individual needs for a sense of orderliness and personal standards for acceptable hygiene and appearance, while meeting environmental expectations that one arrive at work on time and appear neatly dressed to fit the norms of the work setting. These activities occur quite automatically and within a coordinated routine for most people. The skills that are necessary for the motor and mental performances of self-care are organized by habits into a pattern. Thus, a habit functions as collections of performances organized into coherent wholes that serve the larger daily routine.

Habits are developed through a process of mechanization; that is, they become patterned through repetition in consistent environments.[24] Once mechanized, a habit functions as a cybernetic process with the built-in ability to adjust itself within certain parameters. Habits trigger automatic adjustments to allow accomplishment of a goal under varying conditions. As an example, the habit of driving to work allows one to arrive each day although traffic patterns and other factors may vary. Similarly, one can adjust the pace of morning activities of daily living to get to work on time even though one has overslept. Habits of meal preparation allow a homemaker to cook food while simultaneously giving children attention. Habits are like beacons that always return the person to the task at hand and allow it to flow in an organized manner even with a fair amount of variation.

Habits are able to guide behavior in this way because they possess a "canon of rules."[24] These rules, which are not conscious processes, constantly monitor action and make needed adjustments. Thus, the rules must contain information about the goal and about how action can be varied yet still maintain its goal-oriented character. Learned through trial and error, rules eventually become encoded and fade out of consciousness as one practices the behavior. A rough indicator of how much one is functioning in a habitual manner is the degree of attention that must be paid to what one is doing. We all routinely drive to work, dress ourselves, and clean house while engaging in fantasy, thinking about some other activity, or actually doing something else like carrying on a conversation. When we are not consciously in charge of our activities, our habits are.

Habits develop with input from the environment in terms of social expectations and feedback from one's behavior. When these habits no longer suffice to meet the demands of either the environment or the individual's values and roles, then the individual explores new patterns of behavior. As these innovations are adopted by the individual, they become integrated into his or her personal network of habits.[24]

PERSON-ENVIRONMENT INTERACTION

Early occupational therapists asserted that people with emotional problems had succumbed to their stressful environments and that restoration of function was a process of designing and exposing the patient to healthy environments. Modern occupational therapy writers have contributed to a more systematic understanding of how environments influence and shape behavior. Dunning[12] identified three environmental variables as having an important impact on behavior: space, people, and tasks. She notes that an individual's behavior is as much a function of these environmental characteristics as it is of the internal makeup of the individual.[12] Understanding order in the person thus involves understanding how the environment supports and elicits orderly behavior.

Space is a critical dimension of the environment, including both the amount and quality of space available, as well as the placement or arrangement of objects within space. These variables may determine the kinds of behaviors in which a person engages. For instance, a large environment may invite gross motor activity, whereas a smaller one may demand sedentary behavior.

Placement of objects in space can encourage or discourage interaction. People in the environment also use space in recognizable ways and influence others' use of space. Proxemics, or the way people place themselves in respect to each other, includes a culturally learned set of behaviors. For example, different physical distances between people are culturally recognized as appropriate for various types of interactions—thus, one generally stands farther away from a stranger than from an acquaintance and closer to an intimate friend.

The social environment comprises people, the roles they fill, and the network of relationships between them. The social environment therefore influences behavior through the organizing effects of roles, through the collective values of people in the environment, and through the unfilled roles left for newcomers.[1,16,18] Finally, the task environment, which includes demands for task performance, nonhuman objects and their expected patterns of use, and situations that stimulate task performance influences behavior.[1,12,38]

The interaction of humans as open systems with the physical and social environment suggests two stages: a choice or decision to enter a setting and a period of occupying or performing within a setting.[1]

Entering Environments

The decision to enter an environment is influenced by the environment's potential for arousal, interest, and value.[1] Optimal arousal, or excitement, is experienced as pleasurable; thus, environments that provide the right levels of arousal invite one's participation and entry. Three kinds of variables can evoke arousal: psychophysical variables, such as the intensity of color or sound; ecological variables, which refer to the significance of a stimuli to well-being; and collative variables, which are comparisons or discrepancies that arise in the environment or between the environment and the person. The latter category includes complexity, novelty, surprise, incongruity, and ambiguity. As these variables suggest, the impact of the environment is always a function of the person's internal makeup. What is arousing to one person may not be to another person or may not be at a later time when the environmental stimulus is no longer threatening or novel. When the environment provides correct amounts of stimulation, the individual will be motivated to enter, rather than avoid, an environmental setting.

In addition to embodying a potential for arousal, the environment has different capacities to evoke interest.[1] Objects and events within the environment may stimulate interest. Interest exists when the individual sees the potential for engaging in some behavior that he or she knows to be pleasurable or that appears to hold promise of yielding satisfaction. Obviously, different people find different settings more or less interesting.

31

Environments are also sources of different values.[1] Values can be communicated explicitly through verbal or written messages or implicitly through dress, attitudes, types of interactions, and so on. As with interests, settings tend to attract those people who find the environmental characteristics congruent with their own values. Occupational choice is strongly influenced by a person's tendency to see a match between the interests and values embodied by the occupational setting and his or her own interests and values.

It is critical that people enter settings based on choices motivated by arousal, interest, and value.[1] When people do not choose the settings they enter (e.g., when forced to relocate or to remain in a setting), they suffer adverse psychological and sometimes physical effects. Thus, the process of choosing the environments in which one behaves is important for health.

Interaction with the Environment

Once a person has made the decision to enter environments, the ensuing interaction tends to shape both the environment and the person. Press, population density, and objects are three variables that affect the quality and quantity of interaction.[1] *Press* refers to the demands that the environment places on the individual for behavior. Press may be physical (e.g., tennis courts and theaters invite different behaviors by virtue of their physical arrangement). Press can also be social, as when members in a setting encourage or demand certain behaviors of an individual who wishes to remain in the setting.

Population density affects behavior by determining the ratio of people to tasks in the environment. This characteristic is referred to as the "manning level" of an environment. Environments that are overmanned (too many people and too few tasks) offer less opportunity for active participation, whereas undermanned environments provide more opportunity and will draw people into more central and responsible roles.

Finally, the availability and quality of *objects* in the environment determine what kinds of interactions can take place. This has been demonstrated in studies of childhood play where different amounts and types of objects were shown to have effects on the duration and types of play behavior. Objects can influence behavior both through the potentials for action they represent and through the use-expectations they connote. An example of the latter is that a tricycle invites sitting and pedaling in order to locomote, and a magazine suggests reading. Some objects invite social participation, while others invite solitary activity. Some offer opportunity for prolonged but specific activity, whereas others are open to multiple kinds of behavior.

It was noted earlier that the impact of the environment is influenced by the person's internal makeup. Barris[1] refers to this as resonation; that is, the characteristics of person and environment interact to determine how the environment's qualities will influence the person.

In healthy people, the interaction with the environment involves a trajectory of increasing competency.[1] This means that as a person becomes more capable, he or she increasingly enters more and more environments, requires more stimuli for arousal, and can respond to greater environmental demands. Thus, the interaction between the person and the environment is a dynamic process involving a spiral of change.

OCCUPATIONAL PERFORMANCE COMPONENTS

Occupational therapy has always recognized that competent behavior requires the integrity of certain performance components. However, the ways in which performance components have been delineated has varied. These components, which can include such variables as cognitive functioning and motor performance, are sometimes equated with skills or abilities to accomplish tasks. At other times they are equated with the underlying constitutents of skills, for example, integrity of the nervous system.

A Taxonomy of Skills

Different collections of skills and their components have also been offered in the literature, however, no consistent conceptualization has emerged. Some authors offer a wide range of skills, including derivations from the psychoanalytic tradition[30,35] that are not relevant to occupation. To be consistent with the view of order and disorder that has been identified so far, occupational performance components should focus on the skills and their constituents that are necessary for and developed by occupation in everyday life.

More recent works identify the following as occupational performance components: sensory integration, motor function, cognitive function, psychological function, and social function.[8,36] This taxonomy is more relevant to occupational functioning and helps clarify the field's domain of concern.

A recent taxonomy attempts to differentiate between skills and their underlying constituents.[23] Three types of skills are identified as comprising occupational behavior: communication/interaction skills, process skills, and perceptual-motor skills. Communication/interaction skills are those skills employed when one interacts with others and engages in collaborative and competitive activities. Process skills are skills used for dealing with events and functions in everyday life. They involve planning, problem solving, and similar cognitive performances that organize action in time and space. Perceptual-motor skills refer to abilities to interpret sensory data and move one's body in response to and in order to act on the environment. Perceptual-motor skills range from simple perceptions and movements to complicated tool use abilities. These three areas of skill are intended to delineate the ways in which persons act on their environment and the people, events, and objects within it.

Skills are defined as sets of subroutines or constituents that are organized together and achieve some end under varying conditions.[25,33,41,42,51] Thus, skills are flexible routines of behavior that can respond to environmental variation. They are guided by a purpose or intention, and they involve the organized contributions of subroutines or constituents. The fact that skills are guided by intentions links them to the decision-making and intrinsic motivation characteristics of humans. Humans intend action and its consequences when they choose to act for the pursuit of an interest, value, or goal. In this way, skilled action is always purposeful.

Constituents of Skills

The other dimension of this taxonomy concerns the constituents of skills. Three constituents of skill—symbolic, neurological, and kinesiological—make up a hierarchy with the symbolic as the highest level and the kinesiological as the lowest level.[23] Symbolic constituents of skills refer to the internal images that coordinate and interpret incoming sensory information; formulate internal ideas, intentions and plans of action; and trigger and guide nervous system activity.[22] These symbols are internal maps of external reality that inform the individual about the potential for and the constraints on action.[41,42] Images for how to perform skilled action are generated through experience. Human beings are endowed with very few skills at birth, and they must engage in a long period of activity or doing (an open system process) to generate the symbols that eventually serve as throughput in the human open system. The symbols one has acquired serve as internal guides to interpreting intake and formulating output. Thus, they are critical for all kinds of performance. Images are initially conscious and later become automatic. For instance, in first learning to walk or ride a bicycle, a person must consciously concentrate on the intended performance and the coordination of actions. Once mastered, the activity is accomplished automatically, guided by images that are out of awareness. The same process of conscious learning becoming automatic takes place in both process and communication/interaction skills. Such experiences as learning the rules in a new game or learning to display proper manners in a social gathering are examples of how all skills begin as conscious processes and eventually become automatic.

The neurological constituent of skills is the nervous system and its processes. The nervous system is the infrastructure of the symbolic component.[22] Since the neurological constituent is below the symbolic component in the hierarchy of human function, it is organized by and constrains the symbolic processes.

If the brain is traumatized or lacks proper integration, it limits the symbols that can be learned.[28] By the same token, the brain depends on the formulation of images from experience to guide its process of integrated and coordinated action. The two are thus mutually dependent and influence each other in reciprocal ways.

The musculoskeletal constituent includes the anatomical structures and processes involved in movement. Order in the human being requires the coordinated interface of all three constituents and their integration into various skills. The performance of any skill (interaction/communication, perceptual-motor, or process) generally involves an interplay of all three. For instance, communication involves the symbols that underlie language production as well as the neurological commands that evoke motor behavior for talking and gesturing. Similarly, process skills, such as the ability to bake a cake, call on symbolic constituents for the image of how to sequence steps and on the neurological and musculoskeletal constituents for the perceptions and coordinated movements required.

SUMMARY

Human Beings as Open Systems

Open system concepts are aimed at recognizing the complexity of human beings rather than viewing them as simple machines.

Open systems are self-maintaining and self-changing because of a cycle that involves:

1. intake, or the importation of energy and information from the environment;
2. throughput, or the transformation of energy and information into another form and its incorporation in the system's structure and processes;
3. output, or the behavior of the system; and
4. feedback, or information on the process or consequences of output.

Open systems exhibit a primacy of function over structure; that is, the structures of open systems are secondary to and are maintained by underlying processes.

Primacy of function of structure is embodied in the notion that open systems become what they do.

Open systems consist of heirarchically arranged parts. In human behavior the following simple hierarchy is found:

1. the social system
2. the symbolic system (conscious processes)
3. the nervous system (i.e., brain)

4. the musculoskeletal system

In this hierarchy the highest level—social system—governs the symbolic system, the symbolic governs the nervous system, and so forth. Conversely, the lower level systems constrain the higher ones.

The occupational behavior (play and work) of the human being simultaneously calls into play each of these levels and collates them into an organized gestalt.

Intrinsic Motivation

In contrast to motives that lead the organism to seek homeostasis (e.g., hunger), occupation is motivated by a drive for activity.

The motive for occupation is referred to as intrinsic because it proposes that occupation is engaged in for its own sake rather than for extrinsic or secondary rewards.

Intrinsic motivation is the basic drive leading to growth and change in the person.

Intrinsic motivation begins with the exploratory drive of children, transforms developmentally into a competence urge, and finally into a need for achievement.

Actions based on intrinsic motives generate feelings of competence or effectiveness that support and augment it.

Humans as Decision Makers

Human beings are decision makers who must take personal control and determine their own life courses.

Decision making in human life, as it pertains to occupation, is influenced by interests and values, which give meaning to various occupations.

Interests:
- are affective phenomena; they are predispositions to find various objects and occupations pleasurable;
- are influenced by family socialization and social approval;
- reflect an individual's self-perceptions;
- guide choices for action and maintain persistence in action.

Values:
- reflect the individual's cultural background;
- are learned through socialization;
- determined internal priorities of action and lead to the formation of goals;
- specify what is good, right, or important and determine the meaningfulness of many activities;

- have a strong affective component—that is, they carry a sense of obligation and provide a sense of belonging to a group.

Occupational Choice:
- is the major developmental process of decision making relevant to occupation;
- occurs from childhood to early adulthood in series of fantasy, tentative, and realistic periods;
- is a process of optimizing one's inner desires and abilities against a background of environmental supports and constraints.

Role as an Organizer of Behavior

Roles are positions in society that have both status and expectations for performance.

Roles have an internal component of self-experience and an external component of social status and behavior expectations.

The internalized role is incorporated into the person's self-concept and serves as a framework for action; it includes:

1. perceived incumbency, or the belief that one is in the role;
2. internalized expectations, or the perception of the expected behaviors that go with a personal role;
3. role balance, or the healthy integration of roles.

Roles organize behavior by prescribing time use, norms for behavior, and standards of competency.

Occupational development involves a succession of roles referred to as the occupational career.

Role acquisition is a complex open system process involving an input of expectancies for performance, a throughput process of selecting priorities for role behavior, and an output of role behavior, followed by feedback, which shapes the person toward meeting role demands.

Movement through a succession of roles is guided by socialization or the process of social expectations coming to influence behavior and identity.

Occupational roles were originally identified as work and play roles but have been expanded to include the following roles, which have productive and active aspects:
- participant in an organization
- hobbiest/amateur
- friend
- family member

- care giver
- home maintainer
- student
- religious participant
- worker
- volunteer

Temporal Adaptation

Awareness and experience of time influences and directs all of human actions.

Humans have an internal awareness of time shaped by the culture and by development and socialization processes.

Human adaptation involves a natural order of daily life as reflected in a balance of work, play, and self-maintenance.

Habit is the critical regulator of human temporal organization.

Habits:
- organize skills into coherent wholes for the routine performance of daily behaviors;
- are developed through a process of mechanization whereby they become more consolidated over time through practice;
- are cybernetic functions that self-regulate once they are triggered into action; the canon of rules in the habit guides it toward the achievement of routine performances and allows it to use feedback to guide behaviors.

Person-Environment Interaction

Environments influence and shape behavior through:
- the placement of objects and people in space and the available space;
- the social network;
- the task demands for performance.

Entering environments is influenced by:
- the degree of stimulation or arousal provided by psychophysical, collative, and ecological variables;
- the values inherent in the environment.

Interaction with the environment is affected by:
- press, or the demands that the environment places on the person to behave;
- population density or the ratio of people to tasks;
- availability and quality of objects in the environment.

The environment's influence on behavior and its ability to affect entry and interaction depend on how environmental characteristics interact with internal characteristics of the person.

Occupational Performance Components

Competent behavior requires the integrity of performance components.

Components can include motor, cognitive, psychological, and social aspects and generally refer either to skills or their constituents.

Skill is a set of subroutines or constituents that are organized together to achieve some intended end under varying conditions.

A taxonomy of skills is offered:

- communication/interaction skills or skills for acting with others;
- process skills or skills for dealing with events (e.g., problem solving and planning);
- motor skills or skills for moving self and objects.

Constitutents of skills are:

- symbolic, or the images that serve as an internal map for acting on and in the world;
- neurological;
- musculoskeletal.

REFERENCES

1. Barris, R. Environmental interactions: An extension of the model of human occupation. *American Journal of Occupational Therapy*, 1982, *36*, 637–644.
2. Black, M. Adolescent role assessment. *American Journal of Occupational Therapy*, 1976, *30*, 73–79.
3. Black, M. The occupational career. *American Journal of Occupational Therapy*, 1976, *30*, 225–228.
4. Borys, S. Implications of interest theory for occupational therapy. *American Journal of Occupational Therapy*, 1974, *28*, 35–38.
5. Boulding, K. General systems theory—The skeleton of science. *General Systems Yearbook*, 1956, *1*, 11–17.
6. Burke, J. P. A clinical perspective on motivation: Pawn versus origin. *American Journal of Occupational Therapy*, 1977, *31*, 254–258.
7. Burke, J. P. Defining occupation: Importing and organizing interdisciplinary knowledge. In G. Kielhofner (Ed.), *Health through occupation: Therapy and practice in occupational therapy*. Philadelphia: F. A. Davis, 1983.
8. Clark, P. N. Human development through occupation: Theoretical frameworks in contemporary occupational therapy practice. Part I. *American Journal of Occupational Therapy*, 1979, *33*, 505–514.

9. Cynkin, S. *Occupational therapy: Toward health through activities*. Boston: Little, Brown, 1979.

10. deRenne-Stephan, C. Imitation: A mechanism of play behavior. *American Journal of Occupational Therapy*, 1980, *34*, 95–102.

11. Diasio, K. Psychiatric occupational therapy: Search for a conceptual framework in light of psychoanalytic ego psychology and learning theory. *American Journal of Occupational Therapy*, 1968, *22*, 400–414.

12. Dunning, H. Environmental occupational therapy. *American Journal of Occupational Therapy*, 1972, *26*, 292–298.

13. Fidler, G., & Fidler, J. Doing and becoming: Purposeful action and self-actualization. *American Journal of Occupational Therapy*, 1978, *32*, 305–310.

14. Florey, L. Intrinsic motivation: The dynamics of occupational therapy. *American Journal of Occupational Therapy*, 1969, *23*, 319–322.

15. Heard, C. Occupational role acquisition: A perspective on the chronically disabled. *American Journal of Occupational Therapy*, 1977, *31*, 243–247.

16. Howe, M., & Briggs, A. Ecological systems model for occupational therapy. *American Journal of Occupational Therapy*, 1982, *36*, 322–327.

17. Johnson, J. A. Consideration of work as therapy in the rehabilitation process. *American Journal of Occupational Therapy*, 1971, *25*, 303–308.

18. Kannegieter, R. Environmental interactions in psychiatric occupational therapy—Some inferences. *American Journal of Occupational Therapy*, 1980, *34*, 715–720.

19. Kielhofner, G. Temporal adaptation: A conceptual framework for occupational therapy. *American Journal of Occupational Therapy*, 1977, *31*, 235–238.

20. Kielhofner, G. General systems therapy: Implications for theory and action in occupational therapy. *American Journal of Occupational Therapy*, 1978, *32*, 637–645.

21. Kielhofner, G. A heritage of activity: Development of theory. *American Journal of Occupational Therapy*, 1982, *36*, 723–730.

22. Kielhofner, G. A paradigm for practice: The hierarchical organization of occupational therapy knowledge. In G. Kielhofner (Ed.), *Health through occupation: Theory and practice in occupational therapy*. Philadelphia: F. A. Davis, 1983.

23. Kielhofner, G., & Barris, R. *Measuring variables in the model of human occupation*. Paper presented at the American Occupational Therapy Association Annual Conference, Philadelphia, 1982.

24. Kielhofner, G., Barris, R., & Watts, J. Habits and habit dysfunction: A clinical perspective for psychosocial occupational therapy. *Occupational Therapy in Mental Health*, 1982, *2*, 1–22.

25. Kielhofner, G., & Burke, J. P. A model of human occupation, Part I. Conceptual framework and content. *American Journal of Occupational Therapy*, 1980, *34*, 572–581.
26. Kielhofner, G., & Miyake, S. The therapeutic use of games with mentally retarded adults. *American Journal of Occupational Therapy*, 1981, *35*, 375–382.
27. Klavins, R. Work-play behavior: Cultural influences. *American Journal of Occupational Therapy*, 1972, *26*, 176–179.
28. Lindquist, J., Mack, W., & Parham, D. A synthesis of occupational behavior and sensory integrative concepts in theory and practice, Part 1. Theoretical foundations. *American Journal of Occupational Therapy*, 1982, *36*, 365–374.
29. Lindquist, J., Mack, W., & Parham, D. A synthesis of occupational behavior and sensory integration concepts in theory and practice, Part 2. Clinical applications. *American Journal of Occupational Therapy*, 1982, *36*, 433–437.
30. Llorens, L. Facilitating growth and development: The promise of occupational therapy. *American Journal of Occupational Therapy*, 1970, *24*, 93–101.
31. Matsutsuyu, J. S. The interest checklist. *American Journal of Occupational Therapy*, 1969, *23*, 323–328.
32. Matsutsuyu, J. Occupational behavior—A perspective on work and play. *American Journal of Occupational Therapy*, 1971, *25*, 291–294.
33. Michelman, S. The importance of creative play. *American Journal of Occupational Therapy*, 1972.
34. Moorehead, L. The occupational history. *American Journal of Occupational Therapy*, 1969, *23*, 329–334.
35. Mosey, A. Recapitulation of ontogenesis: A theory for practice of occupational therapy. *American Journal of Occupational Therapy*, 1968, *22*, 426–438.
36. Mosey, A. A model for occupational therapy. *Occupational Therapy in Mental Health*, 1980, *1*, 11–31.
37. Oakley, F. M. *The model of human occupation in psychiatry.* Unpublished master's project, Department of Occupational Therapy, Virginia Commonwealth University, 1982.
38. Parent, L. Effects of a low-stimulus environment on behavior. *American Journal of Occupational Therapy*, 1978, *32*, 19–25.
39. Paulson, C. Juvenile delinquency and occupational choice. *American Journal of Occupational Therapy*, 1980, *34*, 565–571.
40. Reilly, M. Occupational therapy can be one of the great ideas of 20th century medicine. *American Journal of Occupational Therapy*, 1966, *20*, 61–67.

41. Reilly, M. *Play as exploratory learning*. Beverly Hills, Calif.: Sage Publications, 1974.

42. Robinson, A. Play: The arena for acquisition of rules for competent behavior. *American Journal of Occupational Therapy*, 1977, *31*, 248–253.

43. Rogers, J. Order and disorder in medicine and occupational therapy. *American Journal of Occupational Therapy*, 1982, *36*, 29–35.

44. Shannon, P. The work-play model: A basis for occupational therapy programming in psychiatry. *American Journal of Occupational Therapy*, 1970, *24*, 215–218.

45. Shannon, P. D. The adolescent experience. *American Journal of Occupational Therapy*, 1972, *26*, 284–287.

46. Shannon, P. Work-play therapy and the occupational therapy process. *American Journal of Occupational Therapy*, 1972, *26*, 169–172.

47. Smith, M. B. Competence and adaptation. *American Journal of Occupational Therapy*, 1974, *28*, 11–15.

48. Task Force on Target Populations. Report I. *American Journal of Occupational Therapy*, 1974, *28*, 158–163.

49. Vandenberg, B., & Kielhofner, G. Play in evolution, culture and individual adaptation: Implications for therapy. *American Journal of Occupational Therapy*, 1982, *36*, 20–28.

50. von Bertalanffy, L. General system theory and psychiatry. In S. Arietti (Ed.), *American handbook of psychiatry* (Vol. 3). New York: Basic Books, 1969.

51. Watanabe, S. Four concepts basic to the occupational therapy process. *American Journal of Occupational Therapy*, 1968, *22*, 339–444.

52. Webster, P. Occupational role development in the young adult with mild mental retardation. *American Journal of Occupational Therapy*, 1980, *34*, 13–18.

3

The View of Disorder in Occupational Therapy

In occupational therapy order is viewed as the ability to engage in a healthy pattern of occupational behavior; therefore, disorder is recognized when a person does not have such occupational behavior.[43] Two conditions have been proposed as criteria for a lack of healthy occupational behavior.[21] First, if people do not satisfy their urges to explore and master the world in everyday occupation, a dysfunction is recognized. Second, disorder is seen where people cannot meet the requirements of the external world. Healthy occupational behavior represents a balance between inner needs and external requirements. When either or both are not met, disorder is present.

A number of factors may contribute or relate to dysfunctional occupational behavior. For example, people may fail to find meaning or purpose in their work and play; they may lack the performance components necessary for competent behavior; they may have poor habits or values at conflict with society; they may have failed to develop interests or a feeling of personal causation; or they may fail to fulfill role requirements. The source of such problems may be past experiences, poor socialization, environmental stress, or organic factors that affect performance components. In some cases, clinical pathology may have precipitated or contributed to the occupational dysfunction. For example, organic involvement or intellectual limitations may lead to difficulties in occupational performance. The occupational dysfunction may also precipitate a clinical pathology. For example, reactive depressions may have much of their etiology in an imbalanced or purposeless life-style or in the loss of an occupational role. In other cases, it is difficult if not impossible to separate medically defined pathology from the kind of disorder that occupational therapy recognizes. For instance, the schizophrenic person exhibits pathological symptoms such as hallucinations and extreme anxiety and at the same time may show a dearth of interests, poorly formed or contradictory values, a lack of life goals, and disruption of many occupational performance components.

Occupational therapists require a system for classifying dysfunctions of occupational behavior.[22,38,43] Therapists in psychosocial practice typically find that the medical diagnosis gives them some information that is useful to consider in their therapy, but it tells only a limited amount about the status of occupational behavior. Thus, it becomes necessary for the occupational therapist to collect and interpret data that help define occupational dysfunction in a given client. Without a classification system, the data cannot be used to arrive at a delineation of the problem in universal occupational therapy terms.

The present discussion of occupational disorder parallels the categories used to describe order in the previous chapter. Such categories may be a helpful beginning to therapists who want to order their observations of dysfunction and begin to label them in a way that reflects the occupational therapy focus and concern in psychosocial practice.

OPEN SYSTEM DYSFUNCTION

The open system maintains and changes itself through a cycle in which the output or action of the system yields feedback into the cycle. Dysfunction in the open system occurs when the basic cycle is interrupted, especially when the action or output of the system demonstrates extremes of activity or inactivity.

In early occupational therapy, central problems in psychosocial dysfunction were identified as idleness and unbalanced behavior. In open system concepts, idleness is a cessation of the basic cycle of the open system.

The Fidlers[13] summarize this perspective in the statement, "A reduction in doing generates pathology" (p. 309). For example, when "action does not follow thought, perception is distorted and the critical learning that comes from confronting the consequences of an act is precluded" (p. 309).[13] Such a condition is parallel to the dissociation of feeling, thinking, and acting in people with schizophrenia. The passive, sedentary life-style of many people may contribute to a breakdown of perceptual-motor and psychological skills. Common problems of those with psychosocial dysfunction—the failure to differentiate reality from fantasy, the breakdown of mechanized patterns of behavior (habits), and the loss of control over one's decision making—are all examples of such system breakdown. Interaction of the system with its environment results in a trajectory of change that can support or threaten adaptation. Maladaptive cycles occur when the system's action is somehow interrupted or disturbed, resulting in a cessation of positive feedback. This negatively influences the person's own internal organization of throughput, further disrupting output. If the maladaptive cycle continues, the result can be total regression.

Insufficient output of the system, as play or work, precludes opportunities for learning the rules of socially competent behavior. A child who does not play may not learn how to engage in role behavior, may not develop physical or social skills, and may not proceed through the fantasy and exploration stages necessary to developing an occupational identity.[32,40,42] For adults, work is both a source of self-esteem and a means of fulfilling the requirements of society. Those who do not work in some fashion are at risk of devaluing themselves and being devalued by society.[5,22]

Further, because work organizes one's time in adult life, loss of the work role may promote disorganization of everyday behavior. For instance, at retirement, people may suddenly be left without a major life activity to organize their daily routine, and they may develop psychosocial problems. Because occupation is critical to the maintenance of health and function, a lack or distortion of everyday occupational behavior is a serious component, if not an etiological factor, in psychosocial problems.

DISRUPTION OF INTRINSIC MOTIVATION

The urge to explore and master the environment ordinarily leads to involvement is a succession of lifelong occupations in which the individual achieves success and satisfaction. The person who encounters failures may develop doubts about the efficacy of his or her skills and begin to feel controlled by external factors.[7] Without feelings of efficacy, individuals find it difficult to maintain morale or commitment to their occupations. This breakdown of confidence can lead to the kind of maladaptive cycle described in the previous section.

The literature on people who are mentally ill or mentally retarded reveals that feelings of external control, a sense of helplessness, lack of confidence, and belief that one is not an effective cause are common among these populations.[18,35] Such learned helplessness can also be a concomitant of maladaptive aging,[48] or may be induced through the denial of decision-making opportunities that can occur in institutions.[30,39] Individuals who do not believe they can control their lives or perform competently do not enact their urge to explore and master.

When people cannot act on a fundamental drive for exploration and mastery, they experience pain just as they do when their needs for affection are unmet. Further, a poor self-image or belief in helplessness is a source of suffering.

DYSFUNCTION OF DECISION-MAKING CAPACITY

Values and interests influence how one acts on the urge to explore and master by directing decision making. When people engage in activities that conform to their value system, they experience greater life satisfaction. People with psychosocial dysfunction may often value the same things as members of the mainstream culture but find themselves unable to pursue those values because of internal or environmental constraints.[18,20] When this happens, they may experience stress and despair.

In addition to discrepancies between values and action, people may experience a conflict within their own value system. These discrepancies may lead to problems of inaction or faulty decisions. For instance, a young man experienced a series of emotional breakdowns precipitated by his return to college after successful periods of maintaining a job as a laborer. An occupational history revealed a discrepancy between his own valuation and enjoyment of physical labor and his internalization of his parents' valuing of higher education. Basing his decision to return to college on a value system that conflicted with his own caused excessive stress, and the decision to return to school inevitably ended in a series of failures and hospitalization.

People ordinarily experience meaning in their work and play activities.[11] Psychiatric patients, however, often exhibit a sense of meaninglessness in their lives.[35] They do not find satisfaction, worth, and other values in their work and play. When people cease to experience meaning in their lives, they become immobilized and incapable of making decisions. Such people are unable to find meaning in, for example, the cultural celebrations of holidays and in the world of everyday work. Modern trends such as passive consumer-based leisure and the increasing standardization and compartmentalization of work tend to further rob the individual of access to meaningful occupations[22,51] and, thus, contribute to dysfunctional decision making.

Interests are also important determinants of choices for action. An individual's anticipation of satisfaction in certain occupations and the internal priority of these likes and dislikes leads the person to action. Factors of economics, paucity of experiences, and impoverished environments may suppress the development of interests in special groups such as retarded persons;[18,20] in turn, the lack of interests can then lead to the inability to structure time in a meaningful way.

People who are unable to identify interests and values frequently manifest difficulty in making a commitment to a form of life work.[16,33,37] Since the occupational choice process is critical for the adult's ability to competently perform in and gain satisfaction from fulfilling life roles, a delay or failure in occupational choice often leads to entry into a role by default or through external manipulation by family, professionals, or others. In such cases, the person's chances of a successful occupational career are significantly lessened. People in occupations or vocational experiences they did not choose for themselves are often unable to perform and thus develop a sense of failure that further impedes their smooth transition to an occupational role.[50]

ROLE DYSFUNCTION

Role dysfunction may occur either when personal needs are unmet in a role or when others find the person's performance in a role to be deficient.[21] Further, a "loss of or change in valued personal roles can result in role disorders" (p. 610).[47] Such disorders, which may be precipitated by mental or physical impairment, are more disabling than the original pathological condition that led to the role disorder.[21,47] Psychosocially dysfunctional people are commonly denied access to normal life roles and are cast in deviant or "sick" roles.[8,18,35] Often the roles that are available to them do not provide a sufficient outlet for capacity and interest. Further, because such roles are not valued by society, they are not a source of self-esteem.

People are judged mentally ill when they cannot perform their life roles.[5] Failure to perform life roles is often influenced by poor earlier experiences in which the person has acquired an inadequate sense of what is required for a role or has not learned how to engage in reciprocal role behaviors. Poor role performance can have a cumulative effect, eroding a person's confidence.[33] This is especially true where earlier roles serve as preparation for later roles. For example, the child who is a poor player may be more likely to become a poor student and worker.[21,42]

Periods of role change and role loss are times of risk for role disorders.[19,47] Role changes may require that a person develop new skills, organize time differently, and actualize new values and a new sense of self. People who were competent or marginally competent in a role may become maladaptive when role change occurs, as in the transition from student to worker and worker to retiree. The loss of a life role, naturally or traumatically, may also lead to role dysfunction if the individual is unable to replace it with another role. Role loss may occur naturally, as when children leave the home and the parent role ends, or it may be precipitated by disease. Role dysfunctions may occur when people have entered roles that do not sufficiently match their capacities, interests, and values. A clinical example is a schizophrenic woman who entered the homemaker role primarily out of a sense of obligation but did not feel well prepared for this role and did not find it satisfying and interesting. Many of her difficulties in daily performance stemmed from her inability to competently perform the role and from her lack of another life role to provide a balance in her life (i.e., a role that would embody her interests and allow her to perform skills that she had that were more highly developed).[25]

Role dysfunctions may occur when people find themselves in too many roles, or in roles that compete for their time or loyalty or otherwise create disharmony. Such role conflict or role strain can lead to feelings of loss of control, dissatisfaction, and inadequate performance. Most people manage to negotiate and balance role performance in the relevant social systems and to develop schedules of healthy role behavior. However, some people, under the stress of conflicting role expectations, may develop psychosocial problems. A typical example of this is the person who feels that he or she must excel in a professional worker role while continuing to be a model spouse, parent, and homemaker and while maintaining multiple role commitments in neighborhood and community groups. Such people may develop a sense of not performing adequately in any role and experience a lowered self-esteem and feelings of loss of control.

TEMPORAL DYSFUNCTION

Dysfunction of both temporal perspective and temporal organization have been identified in occupational therapy. In some instances, psychosocial pathology may result in a distortion or limitation of temporal perspective. Mental retardation, organic brain lesions, and a diagnosis of schizophrenia have been associated with the inability to perceive and conceive of time.[20,34] Temporal dysfunction among people with psychosocial disorders is primarily a matter of poor socialization, poor learning, and impoverished or deviant life experiences. People who are mentally ill often have a decreased sense of future linked to a sense of hopelessness and associated with lowered present functioning.[34,34] Unlike most cultural members who view themselves as progressing along a temporal continuum, people who are retarded may find themselves either frozen in time or moving backwards to a less satisfying life-style.[20] Lack of success in life careers, overall inactivity, and a dependent status give little reason for or interest in the future.[18,20]

Temporal disorganization is also a typical problem for people with psychosocial dysfunction. Mentally ill patients may demonstrate chaotic patterns of time use, be unable to describe typical days, and be unable to manage their time.[34] Such patients may have failed to develop habits to organize their time use.[19,24]

Another area of temporal dysfunction is the imbalance of life spaces in one's time use.[19,44] People who fail to have either sufficient work or play in their schedules may experience psychosocial problems. Without adequate play, the individual is not relieved from the stress of work and given an opportunity to approach and participate in the cultural value system through celebration and ritual. This may lead to problems of burn-out, alienation, and depression.

How one views time and organizes one's behavior in time is a critical component of adaptation. People whose temporal perspectives and practices do not provide personal satisfaction and meaning or that do not satisfy societal requirements should be recognized as being in a state of temporal dysfunction.

DISORDER IN ENVIRONMENTAL INTERACTIONS

Occupational therapists are concerned with the impact of institutional settings, such as the hospital, as well as community settings on occupational behavior. Hospitalization may contribute to dysfunctional skills and roles, to decreased feelings of personal causation, to a loss of interests, and to disorder in decision making.[14,35,39] The hospital may contribute to the atrophy of work and play skills if the patient is not given an opportunity to practice these skills. In addition, skills that are developed or practiced in a restricted setting such as an institution may become rigidly and inflexibly applied in all situations.[3,23]

A mismatch between an individual's abilities and the demands of the setting will also contribute to maladaptive performance.[3] This mismatch may occur because the environment requires a level of competence that the person does not have, or because the setting demands too little of the person. In either case, the person's affect and performance will be dysfunctional.

Finally, the physical environment, through such factors as the arrangement of chairs, restrictions on activities, or placement of televisions in day rooms, may provide few opportunities for social interaction. Consequently, what is communicated is an expectation for maladaptive behavior rather than for the development of functional occupational behavior.[3]

Other factors that may contribute to a deterioration of role and habit performance include lack of opportunity for patients to engage in work, play, and self-maintenance activities; the lack of appropriate role models, unavailability of suitable peers; disruption from former roles; and lack of sufficient stimulation to perform.[3,14,36,39] Frequently patients are in overmanned situations; that is, there are too few tasks for the number of patients. When this is complicated by the fact that patients' activities may be viewed as inconsequential, patients may feel little or no pressure to perform.[3]

Individual decision making is frequently circumscribed by institutional settings, leading to learned helplessness and decreased feelings of personal causation. The long-term effect of this denial of personal decision making may be increased mortality rates.[15,30,41] Personal causation may be additionally affected by institutions because of their inability to satisfy needs related to the self-esteem of residents.[17,46]

Community settings can also foster dependent behavior, afford little opportunity for decision making, discourage activity and interaction, and lack objects and people that can be resources to residents for work and play activities.[27] Different types of environments have been found to have differential effects on the competence of retarded adults. For example, less structured environments, such as recreation settings, may provide more opportunity for retarded people to assume responsible roles, whereas more structured environments, such as the sheltered workshop, may limit their exercise of capacity.[18]

A study of the environments of mentally ill people found that psychiatric outpatients generally did not choose their residences and that they lived in protected environments characterized by a high degree of conflict. Further, their families were ordinarily not sources of support and affiliation, and economic limitations and personal acquiescence tended to make them vulnerable to environmental conditions.[12]

Environmental variables affecting all types of people with psychosocial disorder are stigma and decreased expectations for performance. Both professionals and others have a tendency to expect trouble and substandard performance from the psychosocially dysfunctional person. These altered expectations often serve as disincentives for normal performance. They communicate that other people lack confidence in the person's ability to perform. The types of performances expected of psychosocially dysfunctional people may be a further source of problems. When tasks are trivial, unstimulating, and undemanding, people are not challenged by their environment. The failure to require behavior of which a person is capable is an important variable in limiting that person's competence. Ultimately, "When a life space is . . . restricted there develops little mastery over one's environment and control over one's life situation" (p. 439).[49]

DISORDERS OF PERFORMANCE COMPONENTS

The most common observation made of those with psychosocial dysfunction is that they lack appropriate skills for interacting with others. Interpersonal relations have long been the major focus of mental health. Occupational therapists are concerned primarily with how inabilities or problems of interacting with others lead to failure or disruption of one's work and play. For instance, Bailey[2] suggests that the primary difficulty of psychiatric patients in work role performance is their inability to produce the social behaviors and interactions that are required as part of job performance. Relating to peers, supervisors, and subordinates, making small talk, and knowing how to dress are types of behaviors that can cause trouble in the work setting. Similarly, retarded people often lack understanding of simple social behaviors, such as taking turns, and they often lack the social skills needed for negotiating interactions in the community.[26]

Both mentally ill and retarded people have also been observed to have

50

deficits in such process skills as problem solving, planning, anticipating consequences, organizing objects in space and sequencing behaviors. Problems in these areas may be exacerbated by impoverished opportunities for learning and by atrophy of skills during periods of disuse (e.g., when people are institutionalized).

Problems in perceptual-motor performance have also been noted among those with psychosocial disorders. Many retarded people have perceptual-motor incapacity associated with brain damage, or more subtle neurological problems such as sensory integrative dysfunctions.[1,28]

Skill deficits are ordinarily accompanied by deficiencies or dysfunctions in the underlying symbolic, neurological, and musculoskeletal constituents. In psychosocial dysfunction the major problems are found in the first of these constituents. Symbols or images underlie all skills, from the simplest motor acts through sophisticated social interactions.[31,40,42] They are internalized maps for how to act in the external world. When the individual has poor play, foiling life experiences, or inadequate socialization, the process of symbol formation may be adversely affected. For example, retarded children may not have learned the images of motion needed for game behavior, adults with psychosocial disorder may have learned inadequate rules of social interaction, and delinquent adolescents may lack acceptable rules for moral conduct.[9,26]

Dysfunction in the neurological component may be structural, such as a chemical imbalance or lesion, or it may be a processing disorder. Occupational therapists have been particularly concerned with the latter since the work of Ayres concerning sensory integrative dysfunction in learning disabled children.[1] Interest in this constituent of performance has grown with King's[28] application to adult schizophrenics. Abnormal postural and movement patterns in chronic schizophrenics are seen as possibly indicating underlying neurological disorder and as a possible manifestation of the inactivity of chronically ill people, especially those who are institutionalized.[4,28,29] Given the hierarchical and open system nature of constituents of performance, it is probable that many factors are involved in the musculoskeletal and motor manifestations found in this group. Occupational therapists have also explored the relationship of sensory integrative dysfunction to retarded people.[6,10,45] Again, the possible contributions of inactivity cannot be discounted as an important potential cause and as a covariate of any neurological dysfunction.

The particular areas of skill dysfunction or of deficits in constituents of skills will, of course, vary with the particular kind of psychosocial dysfunction. Additionally, dysfunction in performance components may or may not be a part of psychosocial dysfunction in a given patient or client. Therapists must avoid focusing only on the performance components and/or their constituents while ignoring other potential problems such as decision-making deficits, temporal dysfunction, and role disorder.

SUMMARY

Open System Dysfunction

Dysfunction occurs in the open system when the basic cycle is disrupted by a reduction or cessation of doing (output).

A lack or reduction of doing can result in:
- breakdown of perceptual-motor and psychological skills;
- disturbance of self-image;
- failure to differentiate reality from fantasy;
- breakdown of habits;
- loss of control over decision making.

When the action of the system (output) ceases or is reduced, feedback becomes negative or stops and throughput is disturbed, leading to a cycle that results in maladaptation and regression.

When play is disrupted, the symbols that guide competent action are not generated.

When work is disrupted, self-esteem and social approval for productivity are negatively affected.

Disruption of Intrinsic Motivation

Failures of performance can lead to feelings and images of self as controlled by external factors, without efficacy, and of the future as hopeless.

Negative feelings and images concerning personal effectiveness thwart the urge to explore and master.

Suffering occurs when people do not operationalize their urge to explore and master and when they feel helpless.

Dysfunction of Decision-Making Capacity

People with psychosocial dysfunction may:
- hold mainstream values but find themselves unable to fulfill them;
- have value conflicts (i.e., hold inconsistent values) and oscillate in their decision making;
- fail to find meaning in their work and play and thus become immobilized.

People with psychosocial dysfunction may have deficit discrimination and pursuit of interests because:

- they have been hospitalized and institutionalized and thus robbed of access to interests;
- they have had deficit life experiences and failed to develop interests;
- they may have economic constraints that prevent pursuing interests.

People with psychosocial dysfunction often have difficulty making an occupational choice because:

- choices are forced on them before they can sufficiently develop their own interests, skills, and aspirations;
- they come from deficit environments with limited past experiences.

In the absence of making a good occupational choice, role failure and dissatisfaction are likely.

Role Dysfunction

Role dysfunction:

- occurs when a person fails to meet personal needs or performs the role in a deficit fashion;
- may result from loss or change of roles or when a person is in a deviant role;
- may occur when people are in roles that do not match their interests, values, and capacities.

People with psychosocial dysfunction:

- are often cast in passive or deviant roles;
- are judged mentally ill when they fail to perform their roles.

Temporal Dysfunction

Psychosocial pathology may involve a distortion or limitation of temporal perspective, such as:

- the ability to perceive and conceive of time;
- a decreased sense of the future;
- a lack of self-perception as progressing in time.

Psychosocial pathology may involve a disruption of temporal organization of time use, such as:

- a disorganization of habits of time use;
- an imbalance of work, rest, play, and sleep.

Disorder in Environmental Interactions

Hospitalization may contribute to:

- dysfunctional roles and skills;
- reduced personal causation;
- disorders of decision making.

The physical arrangement of environments may reduce social interaction.

Lack of opportunity to engage in occupational behaviors, lack of role models and suitable peers, and lack of stimulation can lead to reduced performance.

Disruption of roles with institutionalization can lead to further dysfunction.

Institutions tend to take away autonomous decision making and sources of self-esteem.

Environments of people with psychosocial dysfunction are often overprotected, conflictual, and removed from family and the community at large.

Environmental expectations may anticipate poor or deviant behavior from people with psychosocial dysfunction, creating a self-fulfilling prophecy.

Disorders of Performance Components

People with psychosocial dysfunctions typically lack appropriate skills for interacting/communicating with others.

People with psychosocial dysfunctions often have deficits in process skills due to impoverished opportunities for learning.

Problems with perceptual-motor skills may be present in people with psychosocial dysfunction.

The symbolic constituents of skills are images that guide behavior, and they may be deficit in people with psychosocial dysfunction because of inadequate or poor past experience.

There may be deficits or disorganization in the neurological component of skill.

Problems in the musculoskeletal component are fewer and secondary to symbolic and neurological problems.

REFERENCES

1. Ayres, J. *Sensory integration and learning disorders*. Los Angeles: Western Psychological Services, 1972.
2. Bailey, D. A work program in psychiatry. *American Journal of Occupational Therapy*, 1968, *22*, 311–318.
3. Barris, R. Environmental interactions: An extension of the model of human occupation. *American Journal of Occupational Therapy*, 1982, *36*, 637–644.
4. Beck, M. A., & Callahan, D. K. Impact of institutionalization on the posture of chronic schizophrenic patients. *American Journal of Occupational Therapy*, 1980, *34*, 332–335.

5. Black, M. The occupational career. *American Journal of Occupational Therapy*, 1976, *30*, 225–228.
6. Bright, T., Bittick, K., & Fleeman, B. Reduction of self-injurious behavior using sensory integrative techniques. *American Journal of Occupational Therapy*, 1981, *35*, 167–172.
7. Burke, J. P. A clinical perspective on motivation: Pawn versus origin. *American Journal of Occupational Therapy*, 1977, *31*, 254–258.
8. Burke, J. P., Miyake, S., Kielhofner, G., & Barris, R. The demystification of health care and demise of the sick role: Implications for occupational therapy. In G. Kielhofner (Ed.), *Health through occupation: Theory and practice in occupational therapy*. Philadelphia: F. A. Davis, 1983.
9. Carey, C. *Games: An occupational therapy treatment mode for juvenile delinquent boys*. Unpublished master's project, Department of Occupational Therapy, Virginia Commonwealth University, 1981.
10. Clark, F. A., Miller, L. R., Thomas, J. A., Kucherawy, D. A., & Azen, S. P. A comparison of operant and sensory integrative methods on developmental parameters in profoundly retarded adults. *American Journal of Occupational Therapy*, 1978, *32*, 86–92.
11. Cynkin, S. *Occupational therapy: Toward health through activities*. Boston: Little, Brown, 1979.
12. Dunning, H. Environmental occupational therapy. *American Journal of Occupational Therapy*, 1972, *26*, 292–298.
13. Fidler, G., & Fidler, J. Doing and becoming: Purposeful action and self-actualization. *American Journal of Occupational Therapy*, 1978, *32*, 305–310.
14. Gray, M. Effects of hospitalization on work-play behavior. *American Journal of Occupational Therapy*, 1972, *26*, 180–185.
15. Hasselkus, B. R. Relocation stress and the elderly. *American Journal of Occupational Therapy*, 1978, *32*, 631–636.
16. Heard, C. Occupational role acquisition: A perspective on the chronically disabled. *American Journal of Occupational Therapy*, 1977, *31*, 243–247.
17. Kannegieter, R. Environmental interactions in psychiatric occupational therapy—Some inferences. *American Journal of Occupational Therapy*, 1980, *34*, 714–720.
18. Kavanagh, M. *Person-environment interaction: The model of human occupation applied to mentally retarded adults*. Unpublished master's project, Department of Occupational Therapy, Virginia Commonwealth University, 1982.
19. Kielhofner, G. Temporal adaptation: A conceptual framework for oc-

cupational therapy. *American Journal of Occupational Therapy*, 1977, *31*, 235–238.

20. Kielhofner, G. The temporal dimension in the lives of retarded adults: A problem of interaction and intervention. *American Journal of Occupational Therapy*, 1979, *33*, 161–168.

21. Kielhofner, G. A model of human occupation, Part 3. Benign and vicious cycles. *American Journal of Occupational Therapy*, 1980, *34*, 731–737.

22. Kielhofner, G. A paradigm for practice: The hierarchical organization of occupational therapy knowledge. In G. Kielhofner (Ed.), *Health through occupation: Theory and practice in occupational therapy*. Philadelphia: F. A. Davis, 1983.

23. Kielhofner, G., Barris, R., Bauer, D., Shoestock, B., & Walker, L. The play of hospitalized and non-hospitalized children. *American Journal of Occupational Therapy*, in press.

24. Kielhofner, G., Barris, R., & Watts, J. Habits and habit dysfunction: A clinical perspective for psychosocial occupational therapy. *Occupational Therapy in Mental Health*, 1982, *2*, 1–22.

25. Kielhofner, G., Burke, J. P., & Igi, C. H. A model of human occupation, Part 4. Assessment and intervention. *American Journal of Occupational Therapy*, 1980, *34*, 777–788.

26. Kielhofner, G., & Miyake, S. The therapeutic use of games with mentally retarded adults. *American Journal of Occupational Therapy*, 1981, *35*, 375–382.

27. Kielhofner, G., & Miyake, S. Rose-colored lenses for clinical practice: From a deficit to a competence model in assessment and intervention. In G. Kielhofner (Ed.), *Health through occupation: Theory and practice in occupational therapy*. Philadelphia: F. A. Davis, 1983.

28. King, L. J. A sensory-integrative approach to schizophrenia. *American Journal of Occupational Therapy*, 1974, *28*, 529–536.

29. Lindquist, J. Activity and vestibular function in chronic schizophrenia. *Occupational Therapy Journal of Research*, 1981, *1*, 56–69.

30. Magill, J., & Vargo, J. Helplessness, hope and the occupational therapist. *Canadian Journal of Occupational Therapy*, 1977, *44*, 65–69.

31. Matsutsuyu, J. Occupational behavior—A perspective on work and play. *American Journal of Occupational Therapy*, 1971, *25*, 291–294.

32. Michelman, S. Play and the deficit child. In M. Reilly (Ed.), *Play as exploratory learning*. Beverly Hills, Calif.: Sage Publications, 1974.

33. Moorehead, L. The occupational history. *American Journal of Occupational Therapy*, 1969, *23*, 329–334.

34. Neville, A. Temporal adaptation: Application with short-term psychiatric patients. *American Journal of Occupational Therapy*, 1980, *34*, 328–331.

35. Oakley, F. M. *The model of human occupation in psychiatry.* Unpublished master's project, Department of Occupational Therapy, Virginia Commonwealth University, 1982.

36. Parent, L. Effects of low-stimulus environment on behavior. *American Journal of Occupational Therapy,* 1978, *32,* 19–25.

37. Paulson, C. Juvenile delinquency and occupational choice. *American Journal of Occupational Therapy,* 1980, *34,* 565–571.

38. Reilly, M. Occupational therapy can be one of the great ideas of 20th century medicine. *American Journal of Occupational Therapy,* 1962, *16,* 1–9.

39. Reilly, M. A psychiatric occupational therapy program as a teaching model. *American Journal of Occupational Therapy,* 1966, *20,* 61–67.

40. Reilly, M. *Play as exploratory learning.* Beverly Hills, Calif.: Sage Publications, 1974.

41. Riopel, N. J. *An examination of the occupational behavior and life satisfaction of the elderly.* Unpublished master's thesis, Medical College of Virginia, Virginia Commonwealth University, 1982.

42. Robinson, A. Play: The arena for acquisition of rules for competent behavior. *American Journal of Occupational Therapy,* 1977, *31,* 248–253.

43. Rogers, J. Order and disorder in medicine and occupational therapy. *American Journal of Occupational Therapy,* 1982, *36,* 29–35.

44. Shannon, P. Work-play theory and the occupational therapy process. *American Journal of Occupational Therapy,* 1972, *26,* 169–172.

45. Shuer, J., Clark, F., & Azen, S. P. Vestibular function in mildly mentally retarded adults. *American Journal of Occupational Therapy,* 1980, *34,* 664–670.

46. Tickle, L. S., & Yerxa, E. J. Need satisfaction of older persons living in the community and in institutions, Part I. The environment. *American Journal of Occupational Therapy,* 1981, *35,* 644–649.

47. Versluys, H. P. The remediation of role disorders through focused group work. *American Journal of Occupational Therapy,* 1980, *34,* 609–614.

48. Watts, J., & Barris, R. *Aging, the environment, and the model of human occupation.* Richmond: Virginia Commonwealth University, 1981. (Audiovisual presentation)

49. Watanabe, S. Four concepts basic to the occupational therapy process. *American Journal of Occupational Therapy,* 1968, *22,* 339–444.

50. Webster, P. Occupational role development in the young adult with mild mental retardation. *American Journal of Occupational Therapy,* 1980, *34,* 13–18.

51. Yerxa, E. Occupational therapy's role in creating a future climate of caring. *American Journal of Occupational Therapy,* 1980, *34,* 529–534.

4

Action Implications: The Process of Restoring Order in Occupational Therapy

The action implications of occupational therapy are multifaceted. However, they focus on a singular process of restoring and/or maintaining order in occupational behavior through facilitating people's engagement in occupation. This discussion of action implications is divided into four sections. The first section describes the occupational therapy process; the second section provides a list of principles of practice; the third examines evaluation; and the fourth highlights the treatment approaches used in psychosocial occupational therapy.

THE OCCUPATIONAL THERAPY PROCESS

Occupational therapy is a process of gathering information about people and situations, analyzing and interpreting that information, and formulating a rational course of action and a means of evaluating its outcomes. Each of these activities can be delineated as separate phases of therapy: screening and evaluation, treatment planning, treatment implementation, and monitoring progress. Although they are described here as a sequence of activities, it should be remembered that they often overlap. For instance, while evaluation generally precedes treatment, it may take place during a treatment session as a therapist observes the person engaging in an activity in order to ascertain strengths and weaknesses.

Screening

While the most traditional route for entry into occupational therapy services is the physician referral, there are many reasons why occupational therapists may need to screen people in order to identify whether they require occupational therapy services. The most notable reason is that not all patients with medical conditions have an occupational dysfunction and not all occupationally dysfunctional persons have medical problems.[114] Thus, the potential routes to occupational therapy in the future may be much more varied than in the past. Already therapists in such nontraditional settings as the school system, residential facilities, and community centers may take responsibility for assessing a person's need for services.

Evaluation

Once a need for occupational therapy has been determined, the therapist engages in an evaluation process. Evaluation has two aspects: (1) the selection and use of appropriate instruments and procedures for gathering data on a person's strengths and weaknesses; and (2) the organization of this data collection under a conceptual framework that guides interpretation of the data and its translation into a treatment plan. Evaluation seeks to determine areas of order and disorder in occupational functioning. By identifying both, the therapist can plan the person's engagement in therapeutic occupations.

While the therapist's conceptual expertise is critical to guiding the formulation of valid and reliable conclusions about areas of function and dysfunction, it is also important that the person be involved as much as possible in this process. When both the therapist and the person being treated agree on the latter's strengths and weaknesses, the therapeutic process is greatly enhanced.

Treatment Planning

The evaluation process is directly connected to the next phase, treatment planning. Based on the identification of areas of function and dysfunction, the therapist draws up a plan of treatment that includes: (1) expected outcomes or goals of therapy; (2) the occupations and other processes to be used as therapy; and (3) the means for monitoring progress toward outcomes or goals. Both long-term and short-term treatment plans are helpful. Long-term plans may include the most global objectives for maintaining function, restoring lost function, and eliciting new areas of function in occupational behavior. Short-term plans may delineate daily or weekly activities in detail. The latter allow for modification of treatment as the person progresses or otherwise changes while still addressing the long-term plans.

Implementation

Implementation of treatment is, of course, the core of occupational therapy. The focus of treatment in occupational therapy is the facilitation or provision of occupations. Engaging in occupation is an open system process that allows generation or restoration of capacity.

Monitoring Progress

Monitoring progress in therapy has two goals. The first is to examine the effectiveness of the therapeutic program in achieving goals. The second is to determine the readiness of an individual for a new phase of therapy, for a change of settings (e.g., discharge), and finally for termination of the occupational therapy service.

Termination

Termination of occupational therapy should reflect the occupational therapist's judgment that the individual has reached the treatment goals or benefited maximally from available therapeutic services. Too often, termination of service is tied to discharge in an acute-oriented health care system, and patients and clients cease to receive services when they most need and can benefit from them. Availability of occupational therapy services in the community is growing, and this should eventually allow for continuity of care beyond periods of hospitalization. This will require a network of therapists in different types of agencies and a system of referral from one occupational therapy service or practitioner to another.

In sum, the occupational therapy process is an interrelated set of activities (see Figure 1) that the therapist carries out to determine and offer the most relevant services and to monitor their effectiveness.

PRINCIPLES OF RESTORING ORDER

Whether or not they are consciously aware of it, therapists employ certain principles in their practice. While there have been attempts to codify principles of practice, they have generally been in the format of concrete guidelines. Our purpose here is to identify principles that link concepts to action.

Principles are guidelines that are logically derived from some philosophical or conceptual framework and that specify general strategies for therapy rather than representing stepwise recipes for action. Thus, they require thoughtful and creative operationalization and application. To emphasize the continuity of these principles with the field's view of order and disorder, they are arranged in the same categories used in previous discussions. Table 1 summarizes these principles (see page 71).

Open System Principles

The fundamental dynamic of the open system is its ability to maintain itself and transform itself through a cycle of processes in which the output or action

Figure 1
The Occupational Therapy Process

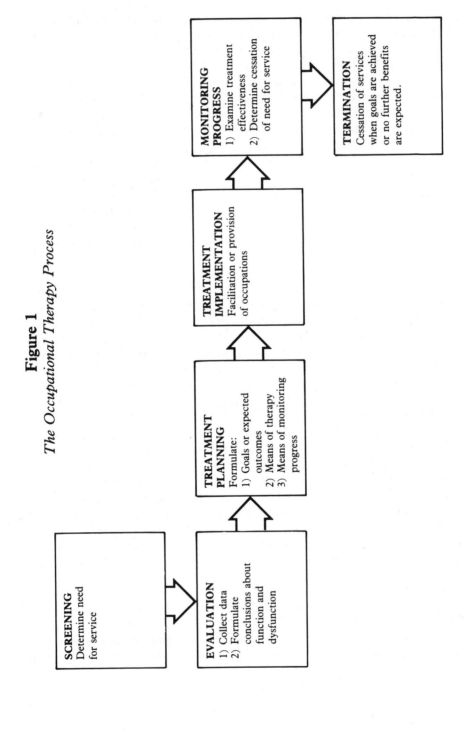

of the system is critical. The open system *becomes* through what it *does*. Occupational therapy is a process of facilitating the action or "doing" of a human system so that it can reorganize, maintain function, and become. The following principles specify how this process is operationalized.

Therapy should seek to increase the patient's productive and playful action.[37,66] A lack or reduction of action signals disruption of the open system cycle. Thus a person's inactivity or passive behavior should always be replaced with action, whether it be simple movement or complex productive activity.

The action elicited should be commensurate with the patient's state of organization or disorganization.[37,66,72] A system's output is limited by the status of the system's internal organization. A severely regressed, disorganized person is not capable of complex behavior and, therefore, should be engaged in activity of which he or she is capable. The therapist should ask what would be a good performance for a person given his or her limitations. For one person it may be the ability to imitate simple motor movements, for another, volunteer work in the community.

Therapeutic occupations should embody the characteristics of normal occupation.[37,72] Occupation is the output of the system and, thus, part of the open system cycle that maintains and changes the system. The kinds of occupations in which a person engages determine the kind of feedback received and eventually what the system becomes. Consequently, occupations used as therapy must represent healthy participation in the culture. When occupations are trivialized or contrived, the person is similarly affected.

Persons must receive adequate feedback on output and its effects.[39,72] Feedback is most meaningful when a person has first determined the goal or purpose of action as a standard to evaluate outcomes. The therapist should carefully monitor people's reactions and verbalizations about performance to make sure they are adequately assessing performance and its consequences.

Increasing levels of performance should be facilitated in therapy.[3,39,62] Reorganization of behavior proceeds from simple to more complex actions. Occupational therapy should provide graded opportunities and demands for increasingly organized behavior. It is especially critical that the environment increase demands as a person's skills increase if new competencies are to be maintained. For instance, one may first learn the method of a craft, later be responsible for managing the supplies and cleanup, and finally teach others the craft.

The reorganizational requirements of the system should determine the kinds of occupations chosen as therapy.[37,68] Disorganization in the human system is manifest in a variety of ways. For a skilled individual whose difficulty is seeing the meaning or worth of his or her behavior, a different course of therapy is indicated from that of the person who lacks basic skills. The output or action of the individual should be aimed at remediating or changing the targeted problem area. In this case, the first person might more profitably engage in values clarification and examination of typical time use, while the second would best benefit from concrete opportunities to learn some new performance or productive act.

Intrinsic Motivation Principles

According to theories of intrinsic motivation, humans have an urge to explore and master the environment. This urge is modified and elaborated through images that people develop of their abilities. People who appear unmotivated do not believe themselves to be effective actors. Restoring intrinsic motivation involves restoring the belief in personal ability and the expectancy of success.

Occupations must be chosen for their intrinisically motivating properties.[16,27,39,71,80] Occupations are intrinsically motivating when the patient engages in the activity for its own sake. The intrinsic value of occupations derives from their relevance to an individual's life situation. A depressed architect plagued with the feeling that she lacks creativity will likely not find a tile trivet particularly meaningful. The housewife who believes she is not a good mother and spouse may not benefit from making something with clay. Individuals' concerns for competence generally revolve around their life roles, and therapy should reflect an appreciation of the demands of these roles.

When people do not initiate action of their own accord, the therapist should exhort them to action.[91] The apathy and hopelessness associated with a loss of belief in personal ability and efficacy can make it impossible for people to initiate action on their own. In such cases, therapists should see to it that they do "get on their feet and do something." Such action coerces the person into a position whereby he or she may "become hopeful by forced exposure to the fact that responding produces reward" (p. 66).[91] Importantly, the message that one is expected to perform also communicates others' belief in one's ability to perform.

People receiving therapy should participate in the process of determining problems and goals for therapy.[3,17,129] A passive, compliant attitude and an expectation of being helped by the ministrations of professionals can reinforce the feeling of external control. People can gain control by participating in the process of designing their own therapy. This is especially important as they progress toward community independence.

The possibility, required efforts, and criteria for success should always be made evident.[16,39] People who chronically expect failure can only begin to expect success if they are shown what steps are necessary and how they can accomplish those steps. Further, by specifying what will constitute criteria of success, the person is enabled to recognize it.

The duration of an activity should be commensurate with the person's ability to maintain a hopeful expectancy of success.[91] People haunted by fear of failure are not able to maintain efforts over long periods. They require immediate feedback on their efforts. Only after a person has generated a series of successful experiences can he or she begin to build on them and generalize an expectation of success to long-term goals and projects.

Occupations should incorporate a moderate degree of risk.[16] Fail-safe projects do not yield a sense of efficacy. Unless the person is aware that a lack of effort or ability would have led to failure, accomplishment has limited significance. The impact of personal effort and skill should be evident.

Decision-Making Principles

The decision to engage in occupations is influenced by an individual's interests and values. Interests are preferences for certain objects, people, and occupations, and values are one's beliefs about what is right and good to do. The ability to recognize personal interests and values is critical to healthy occupational choices throughout life. Therapy often involves a process of enabling people to discover or consolidate their own priorities so that they can become more effective decision makers in their own lives.

Occupational therapy should provide people with the opportunity to discover and develop interests.[12,89,94] Many people come to occupational therapy with deficit past experiences leading to few well-developed interests. Other people come with narrow interest patterns as a result of imbalanced life-styles. Interests arise out of exposure to and participation in situations and occupations. Thus, the action-oriented nature of occupational therapy makes it an ideal setting for generating interests. Further, when people begin to develop interests, they are typically motivated to pursue these interests throughout the day. If the scheduled occupational therapy session is the only time someone can pursue an interest, he or she may be prevented from making natural and healthy choices in the course of the day. Thus, supplies and opportunities for engaging in occupations outside of the clinic space and time should be available.

People should be directed and enabled to develop interests and values that might facilitate correction of past faulty patterns of occupational behavior.[37,80] Sometimes a person's choices for occupation lead to unhealthy patterns of existence. For instance, people may develop only solitary interests, reinforcing a maladaptive pattern of withdrawal from others. Interest and value patterns may reflect imbalanced life-styles such as solely competitive or achievement-oriented interests and values. For example, a group of overachieving, depressed men would need to develop interests and values oriented to leisure and relaxation.

Interests and values consistent with people's everyday settings should be fostered.[3,23,57,68] The development of interests and values serves no purpose if people are unable to pursue them in their life situations. Successful participation in a setting requires that the person assimilate its interests and values. Occupational therapy can increase people's awareness of the values and interests within different kinds of settings. Ultimately, this may lead either to a change in personal interests and values or in the selection of more consistent settings. In either case, when a match is present, competent functioning follows more easily.

People should have an opportunity to discover personally meaningful values by being exposed to a value system in occupational therapy.[6,57,105] People who have been unsuccessful in developing personally meaningful activities and/or a value system that orients them to choices for occupation may come to therapy with a need to develop values. While therapists cannot prescribe or coerce values, they can purposefully embody a set of values in the occupational therapy setting.

Individuals' personal and culturally derived values should be recognized and respected in the treatment process.[38,64,74] People who have been unsuccessful in developing personally meaningful activities and/or a value system that orients them to choices for occupation may come to therapy with a need to develop values. While therapists cannot prescribe or coerce values, they can embody a set of values in the occupational therapy setting. Such values are then present for patients to experience and to make their own choices.

People should be helped to identify ways that they can actualize interests, values, and goals in their lives.[18,23,68,74,102] Some people's problems derive from their difficulty in operationalizing interests, values, and goals in their everyday lives. For example, a lack of skills may prevent someone from pursuing personal interests, values, and goals. Occupational therapy should help individuals to better manage and allocate their time and provide opportunities to develop necessary skills.

Patients should have the opportunity to identify and assess their own occupational choices and to pursue new choices.[68,98,107,131] People may fail to make a realistic occupational choice in the course of development, leading to dissatisfaction and a lack of commitment to major occupational roles. Others may be forced into choices through external pressures or unanticipated changes in life circumstances. Such people may be aided by the opportunity to examine the routes through which they have entered various occupations and careers. If a new or first choice is necessary, occupational therapy can offer an arena in which people begin to match their interests, values, and aptitudes to avenues for productive and satisfying participation in society.

Principles of Role Behavior

Roles are positions in and necessary functions of social groups. When people fill roles, their behavior is influenced by the expectations of the role. They develop an identity that the role provides, and they contribute to the maintenance and development of the social group. Because of their organizing influence on behavior and their importance for personal identity, roles can be used in therapy to influence the process of reorganizing behavior. Roles are acquired through a socialization process that can occur in therapy.

People should have opportunities to enter responsible, active, and productive roles in occupational therapy.[17,127] The "sick" role disenfranchises patients at the risk of making them more helpless. An alternative role in occupational therapy allows people to become responsible contributors to their own self-maintenance and to the maintenance of the ward, clinic, or residential facility.

Occupational therapy should be organized as a socialization process in which expectations for performance are conveyed.[64,110,114] Occupational therapy should be a milieu that embodies the expectation of the culture for productive participation of its members. By participating in this milieu, people become familiar with those expectations and have an opportunity to practice and acquire the role behaviors necessary to fulfill them.

Role behavior is facilitated by participation in groups where roles can be differentiated.[29,37,127] Since roles are the natural components of groups, participation in ongoing groups facilitates their formation and enactment. Groups can also provide an opportunity for people to try on a variety of roles and engage in reciprocal role behaviors. By so doing, they learn the attitudes and responsibilities of members in different roles and how to collaborate with those in other role positions. Enactment of group roles is enhanced when people can identify with a set of tasks and a status that accompany the role position.

Role transition may be precipitated or facilitated in therapy.[52,127] Development involves a succession of life roles. Occupational therapy can facilitate the process of role transition by allowing people opportunities to try out the skills and tasks associated with new roles and to develop confidence that they can fulfill new role demands. In other instances, the occupational therapist may assist people in the process of identifying the need for role change in the present or in the immediate future. Preparing people for the choices that must be made also facilitates role change.

Principles of Temporal Adaptation

Temporality includes an inner sense, perspective, and valuation of time and one's organization of behavior in time. Occupational therapy enables people to achieve temporal adaptation, that is, the organization of daily life behaviors to satisfy one's internal needs and the external expectations of society.

The hospital or other institution should have a schedule of daily activity that approaches or replicates that of the larger culture.[61,110] People who live in care-taking organizations that expose them to schedules at variance with what the adaptive person of the same age would be doing run the risk of losing healthy patterns of adaptive behavior. Effort should be made to establish temporal order that orients residents to the demands of daily life in the community. This includes a time for productivity, a discretionary or leisure period when people can choose behavior, and a time for rest or sleep. At one time, occupational therapists assumed responsibility for scheduling the 24-hour day of the patient. Where that is still feasible, it is certainly within the role of the therapist.

People should be enabled to acquire the temporal perspective of the settings in which they participate.[61,110] Faulty learning, deficient past experiences, and other factors can cause individuals' temporal orientations to be at variance with the settings in which they participate. Some people have not acquired an orientation to the necessity for promptness, organizing behavior in sequences, and discriminating work time from rest time. Consequently, they may not fulfill the demands of various settings. By incorporating the temporal order of the larger culture and the work world, occupational therapy workshops can provide opportunities for people to acquire these perspectives.

People whose past time use has been disorganized or otherwise maladaptive should have an opportunity to examine their temporal behavior, identify areas of needed change, and try out new schedules of time use.[61,79,102,121] This can be accomplished by having people identify how they spend time outside the hospital; classify it according to work, play, or rest; and identify areas of needed change in order to link their schedule to future goals, achieve a balance of time use, and establish a pattern of temporal behavior. This may include a counseling process for people still living in the community who need assistance in planning their time, or it can be a function of discharge planning when people are prepared for return to the community.

People should have opportunities to implement and practice new routines (habits) of time use.[49,65,121] Reorganization of temporal behavior does not occur as a simple function of planning a new schedule. Rather, skills must be developed and skilled behavior must become habituated. Habit change involves four stages: invalidation, or rejection of maladaptive habits; exploration of alternative patterns; innovation, or adopting new routines; and habituation, the integration of a new routine into an individual's existing habit network. Therapy can identify maladaptive habit patterns (invalidation), and provide people with opportunities to try new routines (exploration) and to integrate those routines into a life situation (innovation and habituation). Providing people with opportunities to practice schedules in the treatment context or supporting the practice of these routines in the community are part of the continuum of services that assist temporal adaptation.

Principles of the Environmental Management

The environment consists of people, tasks, and space. Environmental management includes modifications of the task, such as work simplification; modifications to the person (e.g., the use of adaptive equipment); changes in the physical environment, such as the removal or modification of architectural barriers; and structuring or altering the psychosocial climate, particularly through changes in arousal levels and demands for performance.

The environment should provide appropriate levels of arousal (challenge) throughout the treatment process.[3,49,60,64,72,97,110,115] Arousal or challenge is a function of the person's internal status; thus, there is an optimal level of arousal for any person at a given time. When there is too much or too little challenge, a person will not be optimally aroused. As people improve (e.g., as their skills increase), environmental challenges should be increased so that the demands of the environment are commensurate with their abilities.

Opportunities for decision making should be offered in the environment.[3,49,110,128] Denial of opportunities to make choices can lead to learned helplessness and feelings of decreased personal causation. If the overall choice of a setting cannot be made by the person, participation in program decisions, control over one's living space, and optional activities are ways in which the sense of personal efficacy can be enhanced.

The psychosocial atmosphere and the physical environment must be consistent with other expectations for performance.[3,64,97,100] The therapist's actions as a role model, beliefs about the importance of activities used, the physical setting, and objects within a setting all contribute to the psychosocial atmosphere. The accumulated impact of these environmental components communicates certain expectations for behavior. Therapists need to be cognizant of potential inconsistencies between stated therapeutic goals and the environment. For instance, a television set in the day room communicates an expectation for passive, solitary behavior. This may not be congruent, however, with an overall goal of encouraging patients to increase active, social uses of leisure time.

Understaffing the treatment setting can be used as a deliberate strategy to increase individuals' involvement and responsibility.[3,60] People with marginal abilities are more likely to take on passive observer roles when a setting is adequately staffed or overstaffed. In addition, elderly adults are more likely to allow younger or middle-aged adults to fill leadership roles when they are in mixed-age settings. When activities are understaffed, however, individuals feel more personal pressure to assume responsibility and fill positions of leadership.

Individuals must have the opportunity to become involved in a range of settings that increase in their dissimilarity to one another.[3,24,110,113,129] Practice in sequenced, graded settings facilitates the transfer of behavior from one setting to another. However, if these settings remain too similar, the person will be unprepared for the incongruity and unpredictability that occurs in daily life settings. To be truly competent, the person must be effectively involved in a variety of settings.

Principles of Regenerating Performance Components

The components of human performance are one's repertoire of interaction/communication, perceptual-motor, and process skills. They enable one to deal with people, objects, and events. The skills are composed of symbolic, neurological, and musculoskeletal constituents.

Skills are learned best when they have a relationship and relevance to a larger environment.[71,126] Skills are learned in the natural sequence and contexts of daily life where real contingencies and consequences are present. Learning skills out of such contexts can result in rigid or splintered skills, with little ability to generalize outside the learning situation. Further, the development of skills should be attached to a sense of meaning and purpose. Without context, the meaning of skills can be lost. For example, an adolescent hygiene class in which young women put on makeup is more effective if they are dressing up for an occasion such as a dance or outing.

Skills have a developmental sequence that must be acknowledged in therapy.[61,72,90,99,113,125] This principle holds true for all three areas of skills. For instance, play interaction skills develop from parallel, to associative, to cooperative.[86] Process skills develop from the learning of simple sequencing and physical arrangement of action to achieve a task to the complex organization of events in time and space. Perceptual-motor skills begin with simple movement behaviors and proceed toward the more complex performances involved in arts and crafts. An individual must begin with the simpler skills and proceed toward those more complex ones that presume and build on the lower ones.

Skill training should reflect an individual's life roles, interests, and values.[23,66,121] Programs whose aim is to regenerate skills or train people in new skills should recognize that each individual has his or her own skill requirements. These

70

should be ascertained through examination of the individual's life roles and desires for performance. The motivation to learn skills is more readily elicited when this aspect of the person's need for skills is recognized and incorporated into treatment.

All skill training should simultaneously take into consideration the three constituents of skills.[64,72,113] This principle has many implications and applications. First of all, it works both ways in the hierarchy (i.e., recognizing that lower levels constrain and higher levels organize). For instance, if one wanted a patient to organize a skill that involved symbolic awareness, such as planning and executing a craft, it should be ascertained whether the person's neurological and musculoskeletal constituents are sufficiently organized to allow the learning. By the same token, if one wished to achieve better sensory integration at the neurological level, one must stay attuned to the symbolic processes by incorporating motor and sensory experiences into meaningful activities.

Table 1

PRINCIPLES OF RESTORING ORDER

Open System	—Seek to increase playful and productive action.
	—Elicit action commensurate with the patient's state of organization/disorganization.
	—Use occupations that embody characteristics of normal occupation.
	—Provide adequate feedback on output and its effects.
	—Facilitate increasing levels of performance.
	—Use occupations suited to the person's reorganizational requirements.
Intrinsic Motivation	—Choose intrinsically motivating occupations relevant to people's life situations.
	—Allow patients to participate in determining problems and goals for therapy.
	—Exhort passive patients to action.
	—Make evident the required efforts and criteria for success.
	—Choose activities of a duration commensurate with the person's ability to maintain a hopeful expectancy of success.
	—Use occupations with a moderate degree of risk.

(Continued)

Table 1

PRINCIPLES OF RESTORING ORDER

Decision Making
—Provide opportunity to discover and develop interests.
—Facilitate development of new interests and values to correct faulty patterns of occupational behavior.
—Foster interests and values consistent with the person's everyday settings.
—Enable discovery of values by providing a value system in occupational therapy.
—Help people to identify ways to actualize interests, values, and goals in their lives.
—Provide opportunity to identify and assess occupational choices and to pursue new choices.

Role
—Provide opportunities to enter responsible active and productive roles.
—Make expectations for performance clear to facilitate socialization.
—Use groups as a context for performing various roles.
—Use therapy to precipitate or facilitate role transition as appropriate.

Temporal Adaptation
—Provide schedules that replicate time use in the larger culture.
—Enable people to acquire the temporal perspective of their settings.
—Guide people with maladaptive patterns of time use to identify change needs and to develop schedules of time use.
—Provide opportunities to implement and practice new routines (habits) of time use.

Environment
—Provide appropriate levels of arousal (challenge).
—Opportunities for decision making should be present.
—The atmosphere and physical environment must be consistent with expectations for performance.
—Understaff settings to evoke performance.
—Allow performance in a range of settings to increase flexibility of performance.

Table 1

PRINCIPLES OF RESTORING ORDER

Performance *Components*	—Provide skill training relevant to the contexts of daily life.
	—Follow a developmental sequence in skill training.
	—Acknowledge roles, interests, and values in choosing skills to be learned.
	—Consider the symbolic, neurological, and musculoskeletal constituents in regenerating skills.

EVALUATING ORDER AND DISORDER

Occupational therapy begins with careful evaluation of both order and disorder so that therapy can build on a person's strengths and abilities and use these directly in remediating areas of disorder.[114] This aspect of evaluation is critical, since occupational therapy is a treatment process with participation at its core. Without an appreciation of a person's abilities, appropriate therapy cannot be chosen. Further, acknowledging ability as well as disability increases people's feelings of competence.[70]

This section first discusses a number of assessments and evaluation procedures developed in occupational therapy that are appropriate for use with people with psychosocial disorders. Then it examines the process of synthesizing assessment data into a complete evaluation. Problems and issues related to constructing an evaluation battery are discussed and several approaches that have been used in the area of psychosocial dysfunction are described.

Individual assessments yield only pieces of a total picture. Total evaluation enables interpretation of the person's order and disorder. The therapist must engage in a cognitive problem-solving process (often in concert with the patient) to arrive at an explanation of order and disorder. When such an explanation is forthcoming from the evaluation process, treatment can be systematically planned and applied.

Assessments for Data Collection in Occupational Therapy

This section includes a range of published and unpublished instruments, chosen for their compatibility with the view of order and disorder presented in previous chapters. Each instrument is discussed in terms of its relationship to order and disorder (see Table 2, page 81). Presentation of each instrument is brief and designed to help readers decide the potential relevance of the instrument to their practice.

Activity Indices. Nystrom[104] and Gregory[50] developed activity indices applicable to adult populations with psychosocial dysfunction. Nystrom developed a descriptive interview with 61 questions concerning participation in leisure activity and the meaning of leisure. Gregory modified this procedure, constructing a paper-and-pencil self-report in which people indicated their participation in a list of activities and rated them in terms of interest, enjoyability, autonomy, and competence. Both procedures offer data about the degree of activity and positive feelings associated with it. Reliability for these procedures is reasonably good, and both instruments are based on a thorough literature review. Gregory found an association between his instrument and life satisfaction, suggesting that it is a valid measure of activity and the positive emotions associated with it.

Adolescent Role Assessment. Black[7] developed an interview-based rating tool from the literature on child and adolescent behavior. The assessment focuses on role development in the family, at school, and with peers. It includes sections on play experiences, socialization in the family, school performance, peer interactions, occupational choice, and work goals and fantasy. The assessment yields a wide range of data, providing an overview of the individual's occupational development. The instrument has some claim to validity since it was developed from the literature; reliability has not been assessed. Black's own use of the instrument suggests that it can be used to identify patterns of dysfunction in adolescents.

Bay Area Functional Performance Evaluation. Bloomer and Williams[9] developed a standardized instrument to assess the skills that underlie daily living activities. The evaluation consists of a preassessment interview, a task-oriented assessment (sorting shells, bank deposit slip, house floor plan, block design, and draw-a-person) and a social interaction scale. It allows determination of a wide variety of functional parameters, from perceptual-motor behaviors through social interaction. It also yields information on such variables as self-esteem and frustration tolerance. This instrument is supported by substantial research, suggesting good reliability and construct validity. The authors also provide normative data, which enables interpretation of the scores.

Comprehensive Occupational Therapy Evaluation Scale. Brayman, Kirby, Misenheimer, and Short[13] reported an occupational therapy evaluation designed to assess skills in a variety of areas. The 24-item scale is divided into three broad areas: interpersonal behavior, task behavior, and general behavior. The latter category refers to such behaviors as activity level, responsibility, punctuality, and reality orientation. The scale was devised to assess behaviors relevant to and frequently observed in occupational therapy. Each item is rated on a 4-point scale with criteria defined for each rating. The scale was developed to permit efficient evaluation in a short-term setting and to be a means of monitoring progress in therapy. Limited research data support the conclusion that the scale can be a reliable and valid assessment of skills.

Comprehensive Evaluation of Basic Living Skills. Casanova and Ferber[20] developed an evaluation for three groups of basic living skills: (a) personal hygiene; (b) ability for meal preparation, telephone use, and transportation use; and (c) reading, writing, understanding time, math ability, and money management. Each item is rated from 1 to 4 with 4 indicating the highest level of independence. The authors provide no reliability and validity data on the instrument. The range of items appears to make this a comprehensive evaluation, suitable primarily for chronic patients with rather severe skill deficits. However, the evaluation is lengthy and time consuming to administer.

Decision-Making Inventory. Westphal[133] developed an observational inventory for assessing the problem-solving ability of psychiatric patients based on observations of their decision making when they encountered problems in arts and crafts. Therapists observing people in an activity make ratings on a 4-point scale in the areas of finding information, organizing information, and selecting a solution. The items within these areas are based on a theory of the sequences of steps for successful problem solving. The inventory yields an overall score of decision-making (problem-solving) ability and an indication of where in the process the person has the most difficulty.

The advantage of this instrument is that it is one of the few available ways to assess process skills. Further, the therapist observes the person in an actual performance situation rather than at a simulated task. Although it appears to have good interrater reliability, it may have poor test-retest reliability.[28,84] Thus, the user must be cautious not to infer problem-solving capacity from a single observation and should note other possible factors influencing performance, such as the nature of problems, the kind of occupational activity observed, and the individual's motivation. The validity of the instrument rests on Westphal's original assumption that problem solving in arts and crafts is representative of the individual's overall problem-solving abilities. Since this remains to be demonstrated, the main use of the instrument would appear to be as a tool for locating potential problems or strengths in problem solving that could be further observed and evaluated through additional data collection.

Environmental Questionnaire. Dunning[30] developed a semistructured interview designed to assess physical, social, and task environments. The questionnaire yields a wide range of data about the physical environment, such as safety and privacy, autonomy of action permissible, and other related features of the environment. No reliability data are reported. Dunning claims face validity and reports that a pilot study supported the clinical utility of the instrument for assessing the residential environment and identifying areas of needed change.

Home Life Survey. Kavanagh[60] developed the home life survey as part of a study of mentally retarded adults. This survey is based on the concept of behavior settings and assesses the degree of responsibility a person has in the home setting (family or residential setting). It includes four sections: meals, dressing, family activities, and chores. Each section has six statements representing varying levels of responsibility and involvement. The instrument can be filled out by anyone who routinely interacts with the person in the setting; thus, it would be a useful way to assess the individual's home environment and behavior in lieu of a home visit. Although developed for a mentally retarded population, it appears to have wider application in the area of psychosocial dysfunction. Kavanagh reports no reliability data; her approach to validity was to carefully base the instrument on the literature concerning behavior settings.

Interest Checklist. Matsutsuyu[93] introduced an interest checklist in which respondents noted which of 80 items were of casual, strong, or no interest. This paper-and-pencil checklist was originally devised to give information on people's patterns of interests and their ability to discriminate interests. In clinical use, the instrument is often accompanied by an interview to validate responses, discover reasons for interests or their lack, and other relevant information. The instrument can be scored by noting the numbers of strong and casual interests in several categories.

Many modifications of the interest checklist exist; they seek to accomplish a variety of purposes, such as including a better range of interests for certain groups of people and gathering data on past and future interests as well as present ones. Rogers, Weinstein and Figone[16] modified the instrument to yield a more discriminative scoring procedure. Their study indicated that the instrument yields reliable findings, but they questioned the validity of Matsutsuyu's categories as domains of interest. Scaffa[119] developed an alternate form of the interest checklist that asks people to indicate strong, some, or no interest in an activity in the past 10 years and the past month, to note whether or not they currently participate in the activity, and whether they would like to in the future. This version offers a wider range of clinically useful information: patterns of interest lost or gained, the degree to which people act on their interests, and their desires for future participation in interests. Retest reliability of the modified instrument is not known.

Inventory of Depersonalization and Occupational Skill Loss During Hospitalization. Grey[49] developed an observational inventory for assessing the hospital and ward environment and its potential impact on the occupational dysfunction of patients. The instrument examines the impact of hospital or other environments on security, privacy, self-identity, self-esteem, contact with the outside world, and occupational skills. Criteria of hospital conditions and practices that negatively affect these dimensions were used to construct the instrument. The most advantageous use of this instrument would probably be for therapists who are involved in consulting and/or modifying the hospital environment. The instrument also can be modified slightly to be used in residential facilities and other total institutions. Grey reports no reliability or validity data. The instrument was developed from a review of the literature and, thus, has a claim to content validity.

Inventory of Occupational Choice Skills. Shannon[122] developed an inventory of occupational choice skills, a paper-and-pencil self-report of play and chore activities. The instrument is designed for adolescents who are in the first occupational choice development stage. The 29-page item inventory is scored to give an indication of a person's self-discovery, decision making, and work-role experimentation experiences. No normative scores are given; the user is to compare the three scores, looking for potential areas of weakness. No reliability data are available. Shannon used expert judgments of occupational therapists to select and weight the items on this inventory. While both validity and reliability remain to be demonstrated for this tool, it appears to be useful as a means of exploring past experiences with adolescents who are experiencing difficulty in making an occupational choice.

Leisure History. Potts[108] developed an interview for evaluating the historical leisure patterns of emotionally disturbed adults. It is based on a theory of leisure development and employs a semistructured interview format. The instrument yields a developmental profile of a person's leisure experiences and information about present leisure. Potts includes a series of cases that are helpful in illustrating the evaluation and treatment potential of the instrument. She reports no reliability; the instrument is based on a thorough literature review and appears to have content validity. As a clinical tool, it would be most helpful when screening data indicate that a person is experiencing special difficulty in the leisure aspects of adult life.

Occupational History and Occupational Role History. Gathering historical data on a person's occupational behavior over the life span offers information about the history of output and the individual's adaptive or maladaptive cycles. Two instruments have been developed to systematically collect historical data on occupational behavior. Moorhead[98] devised the occupational history, a semistructured interview. It has alternate forms for different major life roles (e.g., worker, housewife, and student, and separate sections for work and play). Analysis of the occupational history involves categorizing data from the interview into the areas of childhood learning and socialization, occupational choice process, experiences of success and failure and their environmental concomitants, and the direction of change over the life span and whether it has contributed to solidification of occupational roles. Thus, the instrument gives data on several of the categories of order and disorder.

Florey and Michelman[41] developed an abbreviated historical interview called the occupational role history. While the content is generally the same, this instrument combines the work and play questions and uses a single format for all interviewees. The instrument is analyzed by examining responses and determining whether the subject is in one of four categories: (a) currently dysfunctional in occupational roles, (b) at risk for future role dysfunction, (c) without occupational dysfunction, or (d) having an imbalance of work and leisure. Their instrument examines the sequence and content of occupational roles, the respondent's awareness of interest and satisfaction in occupational behavior, the organization of occupational roles into a life pattern, weaknesses and strengths in skills, and the balance of occupations.

Published descriptions of both instruments are accompanied by cases that are helpful in illustrating data analysis. As the authors note, understanding of order and disorder in occupation is important background for the therapist using the instruments. Both instruments are accompanied by guidelines that enhance their reliability and validity, although no studies have examined these properties of the instruments.

Occupational Questionnaire. Riopel[112] and Kielhofner developed a tool similar to many existing activity configurations, but with the goal of assessing daily behavior in terms of a theoretical model. The occupational questionnaire asks respondents to report a typical day, noting for each half hour period of waking hours what they are doing. Respondents then rate each activity according to its interest and value, the degree of competence they have for performing the activity, and whether they view it as work, play, or rest. The instrument is based on the model of human occupation (i.e., as a measure of the degree to which the volition subsystem[66] was operationalized in daily life). It indicates the degree to which people do things they like, value, and do well. It also gives information about the balance of work, play, and rest from the respondent's perspective. Data can be analyzed to determine which activities yield the most interest, value, and feeling of competence. It can indicate trouble periods during the day, degree of temporal organization, and other information about daily behavior.

In a preliminary study, the instrument yielded acceptable test-retest reliability and concurrent validity. The advantage of this activity configuration over others is its close link to a theoretical model. This allows a clearer interpretation of the findings of the instrument and facilitates developing treatment plans.

Play History. Takata[125] developed a history interview to ascertain a child's developmental play experiences. The history gathers data in four categories: materials, action, people, and settings relevant to the child's play. It allows the therapist to ascertain the level of the child's most recent play experiences (play development is divided into five epochs from childhood through adolescence) and the quality and quantity of play experiences in past epochs. Menarchek[96] and Behnke[6] revised the play history, developing a more standardized protocol, a scoring procedure, and a guide explaining the purpose of questions and their intended yield. They examined the reliability and validity of the instrument and found good interrater reliability, fair test-retest reliability, and strong evidence to support the validity of the instrument. The play history is a source of information about deficits in these play experiences and settings, thereby indicating areas of needed intervention.

Preschool Play Scale. Knox[76,77] developed this observational tool for assessing the developmental level of children's free play. The scale consists of four dimensions: space management, imitation, participation, and material management. Each of these dimensions is divided into four categories, producing 16 areas of play. The instrument yields scores for each category and dimension and an overall score referred to as the play age. Bledsoe and Shepherd[8] revised the scale and studied its reliability and validity; their findings support the conclusion that the scale offers a stable and valid assessment of the child's developmental level of play.

Prevocational Assessment. Ethridge[33] reported on a prevocational evaluation for psychiatric patients. This rating scale includes three major areas: (a) work skills, habits, and tolerance; (b) socialization and attitude toward others; and (c) personality characteristics. Each item within these categories is rated on a 4-point scale from very poor to excellent. Ethridge studied the scale and found that it was a stable tool (yielding comparable ratings in both occupational therapy and work therapy) and that it was a valid predictor of success in work placement. In addition to its usefulness as a placement and referral tool, research with the scale demonstrated that the occupational therapy setting was just as suitable as work placement to be an observational arena to predict job placement success.

Role Checklist. Oakley[105] developed a paper-and-pencil questionnaire in which people respond to questions about 11 life roles. The respondents indicate whether they have been in, are currently in, or plan to enter each of these roles, and the degree to which they value these roles. Oakley developed the instrument as part of a study of adult psychiatric inpatients, and she examined its reliability in a pilot study, which indicated good test-retest reliability. The instrument has a reasonable claim to face validity since Oakley provides clear definitions on the questionnaire for each role.

This instrument promises to be quite useful in clinical practice as a source of information about the continuity of life roles, future plans for roles, disruption of role behavior, and overall role balance. Oakley described the instrument as useful for creating problem-solving dialogues with patients concerning their own occupational performance.

Sensory Integration Assessments. An assessment of sensory integrative functioning for adult psychiatric patients was reported by Schroeder, Block, Trottier, and Stowell.[124] The assessment consists of a number of motor performances and reflex testing. The goal of the instrument is to provide a comprehensive evaluation of perceptual motor ability. Preliminary data suggest good interrater reliability. Since the authors base the battery on a review of neurological literature and employ many procedures that have already been standardized, it has a reasonable claim to content validity; the authors acknowledge the need for further research to establish construct validity of the measures. The assessment of sensory integrative functioning in children has been widely documented. The Southern California Sensory Integration battery developed by Ayres is supported by considerable research.[1]

Because the sensory integration batteries (both for children and adults) seek to measure underlying neurological deficits, these tests require users to have substantial skills and knowledge. Further, because they are designed to detect and delineate the presence of neurological deficits, they are not appropriate for all populations of psychosocially dysfunctional people. Eventually, further guidelines will have to be developed for screening individuals who merit indepth sensory motor evaluation.

Summary. In this section, a number of occupational therapy evaluations were presented. These evaluations yield various types of information related to the areas of order and disorder discussed earlier which Table 2 summarizes. This section is a general guide to the scope and purpose of the instruments. Determination of how well an instrument evaluates function and dysfunction

Table 2

Occupational Therapy Assessments and Their Relationships to Categories of Order and Disorder

	Occupational Performance Components	Environmental Impact	Temporal Adaptation	Occupational Therapy	Decision Making	Intrinsic Motivation	Open System Functions
Activity Indices							
Adolescent Role Assessment				X	X	X	X
Bay Area Functional Performance Evaluation	X						
Comprehensive Occupational Therapy Evaluation Scale	X						
Comprehensive Evaluation of Basic Living Skills	X						
Decision-Making Inventory	X						
Environmental Questionnaire		X					
Home Life Survey		X					X
Interest Checklist					X	X	
Inventory of Depersonalization and Occupational Skill Loss During Hospitalization		X					
Inventory of Occupational Choice Skills					X	X	
Leisure History							X
Occupational History and Occupational Role History		X	X	X	X	X	X
Occupational Questionnaire			X		X	X	X
Play History	X	X				X	X
Preschool Play Scale	X						X
Prevocational Assessment	X		X			X	
Role Checklist			X		X		X
Sensory Integration Assessment	X						

is ultimately a matter of therapists' responsibility and judgment in any particular treatment setting.

The Evaluation Process: Selecting, Organizing, and Interpreting Instruments

While it is important to know what assessments are available, developing a useful, coherent, and meaningful evaluation process requires use of an organizing framework that guides how one selects instruments, organizes data from them, and interprets the findings. Two types of decisions enter into the organization of an evaluation process: logistic decisions and conceptual decisions. Logistic decisions involve consideration of such factors as case load, the average length of time in the treatment program, the age of the typical patient or client, the ratio of therapists to patients or clients, the scope of the program, and so forth. The therapist must attempt to gather as much data as possible in the framework of available time and energy, while at the same time considering what data are necessary and useful to guide the treatment process.

Conceptual decisions that guide development of an evaluation process involve consideration of the nature of the disorders exhibited by the treatment population. One then selects or constructs a model or some other organizing framework that offers a coherent way of viewing both disorder and the processes of restoring order. By carefully linking assessment data to the variables in the conceptual framework, one discerns the meaning of the data (i.e., what it tells one about order and disorder) and the treatment strategies implied by different findings. There are several ways that this process can be accomplished. The following discussion provides a few examples.

A Case Analysis Method. Cubie and Kaplan[22] developed a system for organizing data on psychiatric patients. The process is guided by 10 analytic questions (see Figure 2) that are based on the model of human occupation.[62,63,66,68] The model incorporates three subsystems: the volition subsystem, which includes values, goals, personal causation, and interests; the habituation subsystem, which includes internalized roles and habits; and the performance subsystem, which includes skills and their constituents. The model provides a coherent schema for explaining order and disorder. Cubie and Kaplan translated components of this model into a sequence of questions that guide both data gathering and assessment. Each question orients the therapist to a variable or process described in the model, and a response indicates function or dysfunction in that aspect of the person's occupational behavior. Attached to each negative response is a treatment strategy. Positive responses direct the therapist to the next analytic question. Thus, as the therapist gathers data

Figure 2

Data Analysis Sequence and Related Treatment Implications⋆

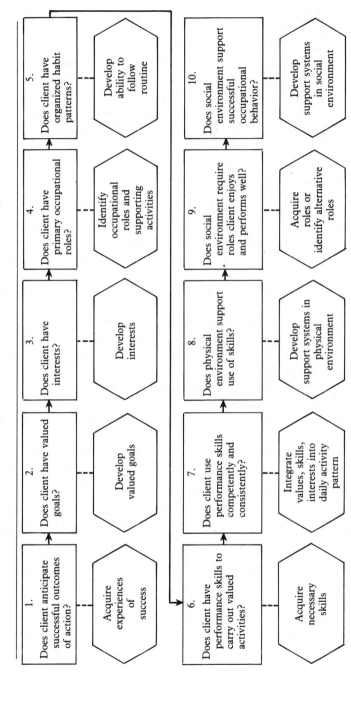

☐ Data Analysis   ◇ Related Treatment Implication

A Case Analysis Method for the Model of Human Occupation, AJOT, S H Cubie, K Kaplan.

The American Occupational Therapy Association, Inc., Copyright holder, Copyright 1982, Vol. 36, No. 10, page 648, Figure 2.

to answer each analytic question, any problem areas that are found are immediately linked to an intervention.

The case analysis process is designed so that it not only allows the therapist to identify areas of function and dysfunction and related treatment, but it also results in determination of the optimal level of treatment. Levels of treatment are based on the model's delineation of levels of motivation and organization in the human system.[62] The lowest exploratory level is for systems at a minimally organized state, and it is aimed at generating skills; the next level, competence, presents greater demands for performance and thus develops habits. At the final level, achievement, the person is prepared for and enters occupational roles. Cubie and Kaplan also identified properties of different treatment groups that qualified them as exploratory, competence, or achievement level groups. By determining the patient's level of organization, one makes systematic decisions about placement in groups. This case analysis method developed by Cubie and Kaplan is an excellent example of linking theory to assessment and assessment to intervention. It provides a coherent approach to clinical reasoning.

A Psychiatric Assessment Battery. Oakley[105] developed an assessment battery based on the same model of human occupation (see Table 3). She reviewed the literature on mental illness to determine which areas of function and dysfunction identified in the model would be critical to assess in psychiatric patients. Based on this, she chose to analyze data on locus of control (one dimension of personal causation), valued goals, temporal orientation, interests, internalized roles, and skills. She assessed locus of control with the Rotter[118] internal-external locus of control scale. Goals were assessed through a questionnaire adapted from Farnham-Diggory.[34] Temporal orientation was determined through the Time Reference Inventory.[117] For the remaining variables, instruments developed by occupational therapists were used. Interests were measured with the Interest Checklist,[93] roles with the Role Checklist developed by Oakley,[105] and skills with portions of the Bay Area Functional Performance Evaluation.[9]

Oakley synthesized the data from these evaluations into an ordinal ranking that reflected the degree of organization or order in the human system. This 5-point scale ranged from very organized to very disorganized, with each level of organization or disorganization carefully defined. In preliminary research the scale turned out to be an excellent index of patients' level of adaptive functioning.

Assessment of Occupational Role Development. Webster[131] developed an assessment battery based on her proposed model of occupational role development. Her model was designed to explain the process of occupational choice

Table 3

Variables and Their Measures

Variable	Operational Definition	Instrument
Locus of control	Self-report of internal versus external sense of control	Rotter Internal-External Locus of Control Scale[118]
Goals	Number of reported goals; number of goals in content areas	Adapted Expectancy Questionnaire[34]
Temporal orientation	Self-report of average number of years projected into the future and into the past	Time Reference Inventory-Shortened Form[117]
Interests	Self-report of intensity of interests	Adapted Interest Checklist[93]
Internalized roles	Self-report of role performance along temporal continuum	Role Checklist[105]
Skills	Observed ability to perform specific tasks	Bay Area Functional Performance Evaluation[9] (shell sort, deposit slip, and house floor plan subtasks)

in retarded young adults. From this model a measurement grid was developed which served as a profile of the person's occupational role development.

The grid profile indicates the status of a person's possession and awareness of abilities, skills and habits, time concepts, values, awareness of values and satisfactions related to occupational roles, interests, leisure activities, peer interaction, family, culture, economic conditions, social status, and social organizations. These variables are identified as critical for the occupational choice process. The instruments Webster used were the Adaptive Behavior Scale[103] (skills); Time Practices Inventory and Temporal Attitude Scale[81] (subtests of a temporal battery used to assess attitudes toward time); the value orientations inventory[75] (awareness of values); the Interest Checklist;[93] the occupational history;[98] the occupational choice questionnaire and pre-work questionnaire[131] (to assess attitudes toward work and how they were learned); and the Work Satisfaction Questionnaire[131] (to assess whether a person can identify job satisfiers). Webster presents a case history to illustrate the use of this battery and how it generated implications for intervention. Her approach is a good example of an evaluation process designed with a particular population in mind.

An Evaluation of Imitation and Play in Children. DeRenne-Stephan[26] developed an evaluation process based on a framework of play and imitation in children. From the literature, she identified critical characteristics of the child, role models, family organization, and physical environment that influence the imitative process in childhood play. Her aim was to examine the young child with psychosocial problems in terms of his or her relationship to the family and relevant environments. She conceptualizes imitation within play as a systems process, influenced both by the internal characteristics of the child (system) and the child's family and home settings (system environment).

The assessment battery (see Table 4) yields data on the child's characteristics and role models, family organization, and physical environment. Each of these dimensions is defined in terms of unsatisfactory, marginal, or satisfactory status, providing criteria for interpreting data from instruments. The overall data collection and analysis process yields a profile of the child's play/imitation status. She illustrates how the determination of the status leads to intervention strategies through the presentation of a case. As with the previous evaluation battery, this one is an example of taking a particular process critical to occupational development in a defined population and developing a conceptual framework and related assessment process.

Assessing the Developmental Level of Play. Lindquist, Mack, and Parham[86,87] developed a model to synthesize the sensory integration performance constituent of skill and play output of the child. They explained how sensory

Table 4

Summary of Relationships Between Imitation Factors and the Instruments

Characteristics of the Child	Instrument
1. Vision	1. Play Scale[76,77] Play History[125]
2. Visual Imagery	2. Imaginative Play Scale[76,77]
3. Skill	3. Play Scale[76,77] Play History[125]

Characteristics of Models	Instrument
1. Degree of competence, status, and control over resources	1. Play History[125] Social Competence Interview
2. Nurturing, rewarding behaviors	2. Child/Parent Observation[26]
3. Contagious, major sources of support and control of resources	3. Social Competence Interview Time Analysis[81]
4. Similarity of model to child	4. Child/Parent Observation[26]
5. Number of models having similar behavior and values	5. Time Analysis[81] Play History[125]
6. Similarity of model to dominant values of mainstream culture	6. Value Orientation Inventory[75] Social Competence Interview Internal-External Scale[118] Play History[125]
7. Observation of consequences for model	7. Child/Parent Observation[26]

Characteristics of Family Organization	Instrument
1. Status	1. Social Competence Interview
2. Value	2. Internal-External Scale[118] Value Orientation Inventory
3. Psychological Outcome	3. Social Competence Interview Time Analysis[81]

Characteristics of Physical Environment	Instrument
1. Play Environment	1. Play Agenda[97] Play History[125]

Imitation: A Mechanism of Play Behavior, AJOT, C deRenne-Stephen.

motor processes intermesh with childhood play and the hierarchical organization of play behavior in development. Like the previous authors, they used a systems framework to organize their concepts of play and sensory integration. Assessment plans were developed for the input and throughput processes at three developmental/hierarchical levels: sensory motor, constructive, and social (see Table 5). The authors identified appropriate historical, observational, and standardized occupational therapy instruments and other measures of play behaviors and underlying sensory motor performance capacity. The meaning and interpretations of the assessments are derived from their hierarchical systems model.

This evaluation procedure is especially significant because it represents a synthesis of both occupational performance components and a concern for the child's role as a player. Both are seen as integrated facets of the child. Their schema is a cogent alternative to assessment approaches that focus on only one element or dimension of childhood function while ignoring other important processes. Further, their assessment battery reflects an appreciation for the hierarchical nature of human order.

Summary

This discussion provided an overview of five approaches to organizing the evaluation process. These approaches provide insight into the importance of systematically constructing evaluation procedures and the care that goes into a well-constructed evaluation battery. Each of these batteries proceeded from an examination of occupational therapy themes relevant to a particular setting or population and a type of occupational behavior. This enabled the identification of useful instruments, as well as a meaningful framework for their interpretation.

THE FUNCTIONS AND PROCESSES OF THE OCCUPATIONAL THERAPIST IN PSYCHOSOCIAL DYSFUNCTION

Occupational therapy facilitates participation in adaptive patterns of occupations to elicit, maintain, or restore order. There are three broad ways in which occupational therapists accomplish this. First, occupational therapists directly engage people in occupations (see Figure 3). Second, occupational therapists collaborate with people to enable them to understand their own maladaptive occupational patterns and to alter them through problem solving, planning, and practice. Third, occupational therapists facilitate engagement in occupations by creating a better match between people and their environments. This can be accomplished by effecting changes in the person (e.g.,

Table 5
Assessments of Play Development Considering Environmental (Input) Factors and Internal Processing (Throughput) Factors*

Development Level of Play

Assessment	Sensory Motor		Constructive		Social	
	Input	Throughput	Input	Throughput	Input	Throughput
History	Play history[125]	Sensory history Play history[125]	Play history[125]	Play history[125]	Play history[125]	Play history[125]
Observation	Play agenda[97]	Play scale[16,77] Reflex, range of motion, spasticity, and muscle testing. Clinical observations	Play agenda[97]	Play scale[76,77] Play observation	Play agenda[97]	Observation of social participation Observation of sociodramatic play—Smilansky
Standardized Test	Home observation of the environment (HOME)	Bayley infant scales Bruininks-Oseretsky Test of Motor Proficiency Gesell test Southern California Sensory Integration Test—Ayres Uzgiris-Hunt scales	HOME	Portions of Bayley, Gesell, Uzgiris-Hunt		

A Synthesis of Occupational Behavior and Sensory Integration Concepts in Theory and Practice, Part 2: Clinical Applications, AJOT, JE Lindquist, W Mack, LD Parham.

The American Occupational Therapy Association, Inc., Copyright holder, Copyright 1982, Vol. 36. No. 7, page 435, Table 1.

Figure 3

The Means by which Occupational Therapists Facilitate Healthy Occupation to Elicit, Restore or Maintain Order

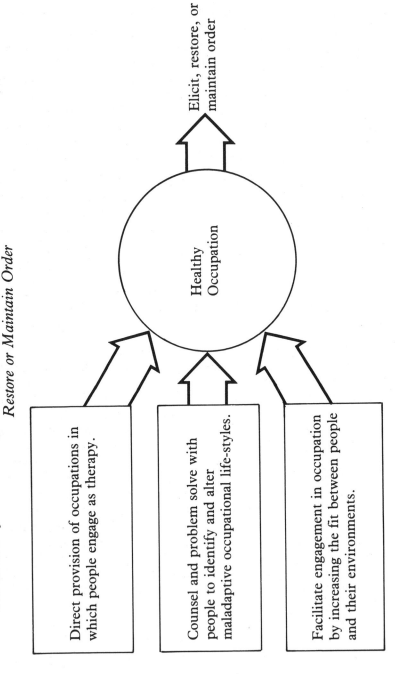

clarifying values, learning new skills) or by altering the environment (e.g., reducing demands, providing structure, increasing resources).

These three broad approaches can be organized into a number of roles and functions of occupational therapists: (1) the therapist as environmental manager, (2) the therapist as mutual problem solver and co-planner, (3) the therapeutic use of self, (4) the use of occupations as therapy, and (5) the use of task-oriented groups. Each of these roles and functions employs concepts of order and disorder.

The Occupational Therapist as Environmental Manager

In moral treatment, the primary therapeutic approach was the arrangement of a healthy environment. The role of the occupational therapist as environmental manager has evolved from this approach.[11] In early occupational therapy, when all patients were treated in the context of the institution, the role was primarily one of making the hospital a healthy place to work and play. With the advent of community-based care and deinstitutionalization, the role of environmental manager became more complex and expanded to include the community. This section first examines the role of the occupational therapist in creating a health-inducing environment, and then discusses the occupational therapist's increasing involvement in community settings.

Creating a Context for Treatment. Early occupational therapists paid considerable attention to the psychosocial environment. In describing occupational therapy programs, writers referred to the mood of cheerfulness and hope, the esprit de corps, the sense of purpose and industry, the feeling of order and rhythm, and other aesthetic and psychosocial properties that exerted a positive influence on the attitudes, conscious processes, and eventual recovery of patients.[67] Bateson[4] argued that occupational therapists must recognize this psychosocial dimension as an essential part of the treatment process. Patient participation in activities is a function of the way in which the environment is organized, the messages given off by the therapist concerning the activity, and the therapist's own attitudes toward the activity. If the activity does not matter a great deal to the therapist, and if the environment does not communicate this concern, the activity becomes a contrivance rather than a genuine human endeavor for the patient. Engelhardt[32] suggested that occupational therapy has as its foundation an appreciation of the value of human achievement and human commerce with the environment and with fellow humans.

Through the communication of such values, occupational therapy has a role in the construction or reconstruction of reality for patients.[123] By becoming a context for action (with certain psychosocial parameters), the occupational therapy setting defines what the patient does and thereby influences how that patient experiences the reality of his or her action and existence. A context is a setting or framework that communicates certain messages and expectations for behavior. The idea of a context or frame is borrowed from our understanding of how such phenomena occur in daily life. For instance, as one enters a church, a classroom, a concert hall, or a romantic French restaurant, it is altogether common to be "moved" by the feeling or tone of the setting and its members, and to feel a compulsion to act in accordance with the implicit rules of conduct. The occupational therapy clinic is not a church or a concert hall, but it is a human context in which the participants will experience and participate in something. By consciously recognizing this fact and carefully arranging the psychosocial climate of the clinic, the therapist has an important impact on what the person will experience and do. Occupational therapists employ identifiable psychosocial contexts derived from the larger culture, such as festivity and ritual, sport, craft, school, and work. Each has its own internal definition and messages, its own mood and meaning, its rules of conduct, and its particular way of influencing the actors within it. Ultimately, occupational therapy provides a context of caring, one that values work and play and signifies hope and the possibility of positive change in the human condition.[134]

A number of sport and game contexts have been used in occupational therapy.[37,56,69] Puzzles provide a sense of mastery over the environment, while games of chance offer events in which one has no such control over outcomes. Games of strategy add a human factor of competition, overt action, and careful attention to others. With each type of game or sport, different behaviors, moods, and values emerge. For example, in games of strategy, fast action and risk in uncertainty may be important values and behaviors. Another type of context that has been used in occupational therapy is that of an educational or school setting.[85] In this context, learning and study are the expected client behaviors. To this end, clients are referred to as students and therapy groups as classes.

The physical and architectural properties of a setting and the dress, behavior, values, and ideals of other people in the setting all help to shape the context. For example, the hospital cafeteria under usual conditions will convey a context of mealtime activities. Transforming the cafeteria with streamers, music, and people in dress clothes who are socializing or dancing communicates a completely different context—that of a party or dance. Work-oriented programs frequently rely on the artifacts and rituals of the real work world to create a simulated work context for clients.[55] For instance, recording members' hours on daily payroll sheets and giving out checks once a week communicate expectations for work behavior similar to that in a real work setting.

Verbal and nonverbal communication also shape the context. When a therapist invites a hospitalized child to "pretend," enjoins a retarded adolescent to take a chance in some game, or joins a group of adult patients in a volunteer program, important messages are given about the expectations, the value, and the possibilities of an activity. Thus, what the therapist communicates by virtue of both talk and action can serve to reinforce or initiate a particular context that is being evoked for therapy.

Anything done to "physically" structure the environment will affect the psychosocial context. Similarly, creating a particular psychosocial atmosphere necessitates corresponding physical changes in the setting. In the previous example of the hospital cafeteria, the context of a holiday dance was enhanced by the use of decorations and other cosmetic changes in the setting. Structuring an activity in a certain way will also influence the psychosocial climate. Providing each member of a group with individual materials and tools communicates expectations for social behavior that are quite different from those communicated by placing a limited number of supplies in the center of a table.[100]

Many occupational therapy interventions contribute to the creation of a general context of competence. One principle for structuring the environment previously noted is that the demands for performance should match the patient's abilities. Essentially, this is the traditional occupational therapy rule of "grading" activities. For instance, in a program of sports with retarded men, sessions progressed from catch to football as the men's athletic prowess increased.[69] In this transition, the environmental demands associated with the games were for increasingly complex levels of skill.

A context for competence is maintained when individuals' feelings of being in control are not undermined by the setting. Involuntary relocation to an institutional setting may infringe on people's sense of control. However, visiting the setting in advance of the actual move, knowing that one's room is a place of privacy, being able to bring one's own possessions and decorations into the room, and continuing contact with friends and activities in the community are environmental interventions that can alleviate the potential feeling of loss of control.[51,128]

Structuring the environment for competence also entails an understanding of which physical conditions are most likely to promote adaptive performance for particular clients. For example, emotionally disturbed children's performance may be enhanced in a distraction-free room with structured activity.[78] For other people, the hospital environment may be understimulating and a more arousing setting may be necessary to induce individuals to give up the passive sick role and resume more active roles.[106]

Managing the environment to create frames for adaptive occupational performance is an intricate and complex process. Everything the therapist says, does, and provides—from interactions with the client to the physical setting, to the choice of activity—is predicated on and contributes to the shaping of the context.

Managing the Community Environment. In the 1950s and 1960s, there was a reverse of the practice of committing psychiatric patients to long-term hospitalization. The community mental health movement has had implications for all mental health workers. In particular, occupational therapists have found themselves modifying and redefining their roles to include more comprehensive responsibility for managing client treatment, to accommodate the changing roles of other disciplines, and to shape a more equal, nonmedical client/therapist relationships.

The role of the occupational therapist as an environmental manager is one that naturally and meaningfully extends into the community.[71,89] Bockoven[10,11] and Ethridge[33] promote the movement of occupational therapists into responsible leadership positions in community mental health programming. They argue that occupational therapists should establish themselves in roles as community organizers, program developers, and administrators.

The nature of work in the community is quite different from that in hospital clinics.[33] The latter is secure and structured, with limited physical borders, familiar administrative structures and co-worker relationships, a degree of orderliness and domination by the medical profession. The community, a nontraditional work setting for occupational therapists, is characterized by less structure, no physical boundaries, new administrative and co-worker relationships, and a relatively nonmedical orientation. In the hospital setting, the therapeutic relationship tends to be more vertical, with the therapist as helper and the client in a dependent patient role. The community is more conducive to horizontal relationships, in which the therapist is a friendly collaborator in guiding the client and enabling greater client independence.

In the community the therapist needs to be familiar with local standards; to work with a wide range of key support people and agencies such as teachers, neighbors, family and friends, and government and social-recreational groups; and to be familiar with work or volunteer opportunities and the range of productive and play activities available in the community. In addition, the community demands a broader understanding of the life situation, culture, history, and environments in which clients exist and act in order to provide optimally meaningful intervention.[71]

Occupational therapists may be found working in residential programs such as group homes for the mentally retarded, halfway houses, club house rehabilitation programs for deinstitutionalized psychiatric patients, and day treatment programs.[25,53,55,88,89] Programs that have been developed to bridge the gap between the hospital and the community and to prevent rehospitalization include quarterway house programs, partial hospitalization, and other transitional programs.[79,80,92,130] Community programs for the well elderly population have been developed as a prevention strategy.[18,73] In these community programs occupational therapists have worked to promote adjustment and independence in their clients through intervention that focuses on the development of a range of life skills, from grooming to job seeking. For example, a work-oriented day care program with a strong occupational therapy component and a temporary employment program emphasized the value of work in terms of the opportunity it offers for meaningful participation in society.[55] Members attending the work component were found to be more self-directed, more active in directing their treatment program, and more hopeful regarding goal achievement than were clients in the general activity program component. The clubhouse model developed by Fountain House in New York City has influenced the design of many community treatment programs for the long-term psychiatric patient. This is a psychosocial rehabilitation model that requires maximal member involvement in maintaining the clubhouse operation. It offers members the opportunity to be either temporary or full-time workers in competitive employment. The program includes a clubhouse, temporary employment program, apartment program, and various other components. Members' attendance at the clubhouse is wanted, expected, and needed for clubhouse functioning. The model is based on the beliefs that even the most severely psychosocially dysfunctional person can be productive, that work is a worthwhile "regenerative and reintegrative" goal, and that recreational and social activities have value in the normal daily routine.[5]

Transitional programs are designed to ease the move from hospital to community. One task-oriented daily living group available to predischarge patients focused on the use of leisure time, learning about community resources, and general problem solving related to the discharge process.[53] Another, a quarterway house program developed by occupational therapists on the grounds of a state hospital, allowed patients to take increased responsibility in preparation for their return to the community.[92]

A program called neighborhood extension of activity therapy was designed to aid in transition to the community by promoting use of existing community leisure resources.[79] This program emphasized the exploration and matching of interests and resources to promote client involvement in the community. A different type of community program was developed as a preventive strategy for well elderly participants.[73] Elderly clients attending a nutrition program were given avocational and recreational activities, physical exercises, and educational sessions for the purpose of increasing life satisfaction. Positive changes were noted in clients' levels of socialization, general affect, and life satisfaction.

These programs demonstrate the therapist's role as environmental manager and the variety of uses of the community setting for promoting mental health and life satisfaction and providing meaningful, responsible, and productive roles for people in the community.

Therapist as Co-Problem Solver and Co-Planner

Earlier discussions implied that occupational therapists do not function as one-to-one or group psychotherapists. This issue is often confused with that of the appropriateness of occupational therapists offering counseling as part of therapy. This confusion arises over the mistaken notion that counseling implies a psychotherapeutic approach along with its typical goals of achieving emotional catharsis and insight into intrapsychic dynamics. Quite the contrary, counseling is a process that can have very different goals and purposes and that may be used as part of occupational therapy.

The counseling process should be viewed in light of its intended functions in occupational therapy—that is, facilitating the person's participation in a pattern of healthy occupation. This goal can be addressed in the counseling process when the therapist engages in mutual problem solving and planning with individuals. For instance, people often have problems managing their time, relating activities to goals, and identifying problem areas in their daily life occupations. By helping such individuals achieve new directions, decisions, life plans, and time schedules, the occupational therapist facilitates occupation and health.

Three broad areas of occupational counseling can be differentiated: time management planning and problem solving, leisure counseling, and occupational choice counseling. All aim to actively involve the consumer in identifying problem areas and strengths, goal setting, and planning a course of action.[94]

In occupational therapy, counseling results in action through the setting of a goal for performance, be it a full week's schedule or a single hour of activity. Client performance is thus an essential part of this counseling process. For instance, a therapist offering leisure counseling may have established with a client the goal of attending a dance. In the following session, the therapist and client would explore together what had happened, whether the client's actions were adaptive or maladaptive, and decide whether it is time to go on to another activity, if more practice in the same activity is needed, or some other option. Thus, new goals for task performance are set as an outcome of ongoing performance evaluation.

The goal setting process is essential for all occupational therapy counseling regardless of its focus or whether it occurs in an inpatient or outpatient setting. In time, the client should internalize the process and continue it independently. Thus, the person should eventually be able to get information, make well-informed decisions about personal changes and goals, decide on the appropriate tasks related to those goals, set about doing the tasks, and evaluate their outcomes.

Time Management Planning and Problem Solving. Counseling regarding the healthy use of time is a role of occupational therapists. A framework of temporal adaptation[61] can serve as a guide to time management planning and problem solving. Using it the therapist seeks to gather data on several relevant aspects of the person's temporal adaptation. The therapist initially explores the degree of balance in the person's daily life through a diary self-report of time use, a report of a typical day, or an interview aimed at reconstructing the person's usual daily behavior. Lack of leisure time, insufficient work time, lack of rest or sleep, and disorganized time use can be identified. Importantly, the balance of work, play, rest, and sleep includes not only the amounts of time devoted to each activity but also a qualitative dimension. For instance, a person with a smaller percentage of time devoted to recreation may have a more balanced life-style than someone else who has more time for recreation but who replicates the competitive and achievement oriented nature of work in recreation.

A second critical dimension of evaluation is the relationship between an individual's values, interests, and goals and his or her use of time. The occupational questionnaire can be used to assess the degree to which people enact their interests and values in daily life. A third dimension of temporal adaptation is the degree to which a person's time use reflects a balance of life roles. A therapist can explore whether or not the individual has sufficient numbers of roles to organize time use, whether there is role conflict (i.e., roles presenting conflicting demands for time use), or whether the individual's time use reflects a failure to meet role demands. A further dimension is the match of a person's time use to the environments within which he or she performs. Each setting has its own requirements for how occupants use time, and competence is reflected in a person's ability to meet those requirements.

Another area to be examined is the relationship of temporal patterns to any pathology or limitations of performance. Here, two issues are involved: adjustments that must be made to disease and its constraints, and the impact of patterns of time use on pathological processes. Some people with psychosocial dysfunction have physical limitations (e.g., cerebral palsy) or emotional or mental limitations (e.g., cognitive problems or low stress tolerance) which necessitate schedules that maximize their strengths while taking into account these limitations. For instance, a man who has cerebral palsy, but who wants to appear neatly dressed may spend a great deal of time each morning in self-care. The value of self-care and appearance to this individual make it important to maintain it as part of his schedule. For someone else, trying to pursue two roles, such as worker and student, might produce more stress than the person can tolerate. In this case, it is important to realize that one role may need to be given up if the person is to cope successfully with the other.

The second issue, the impact of time use on pathology, describes a situation in which a person's time use can be identified as directly contributing to a psychosocial problem. One may identify how the overscheduled day of a workaholic contributes to a sense of helplessness and depression or how the chaotic and unplanned day of a schizophrenic contributes to disorientation and a sense of unreality.

The goals of counseling for temporal adaptation are organized along the same dimensions as evaluation. The therapist and client seek to schedule a balanced daily and weekly routine that allows the client time to pursue work, play, and rest; time to fulfill life roles; and time to enact values and interests while meeting the reasonable demands of the environment. Sometimes, this process involves tasks other than simply planning time. Clarifying values, deciding to drop an unnecessary role, negotiating with others for altered role demands, developing skills for more efficient time use, and identifying interests to guide temporal behavior are examples of strategies that might be pursued as part of establishing a healthy use of time in daily life.

One of the most important aspects of time management counseling is helping people achieve an integration between present time use and future goals. By identifying the tasks needed for a future goal and integrating them into the present, the person may achieve a relationship between present patterns of time use and orientation to the future. This often involves the important process of occupational choice, which, because of its complexity, is treated here as a separate area of occupational therapy counseling.

Occupational Choice Counseling. Occupational choice counseling refers to facilitating a lifelong process of choices for occupational roles that may include work, but that extend to many other occupational behaviors. Further, occupational choice refers to much more than the process of identifying and selecting a job or an area of training for work. It involves the developmental process of anticipating success and satisfaction in life occupations, of developing interests, values, and a personal identity. The occupational therapist intervenes when occupational choice is developmentally delayed and when people demonstrate patterns of having made poor choices for occupational behavior. Occupational choice counseling may culminate in referral of an individual to a vocational or rehabilitation counselor who can help a person select training opportunities, identify resources for training, and so on. Finally, because occupational therapists recognize occupational choice as a process involving a dynamic interplay of action, choice, feedback, and further action, they integrate occupational choice counseling with the prescription and planning of experiences, skill training, values clarification procedures, and other processes that facilitate development of occupational choice.

Paulson[107] and Webster[131] offer schemas of occupational choice and of assessing the developmental level of choice. They also illustrate the various action implications of occupational choice problems that serve as a guide to setting up tasks for clients to pursue as part of a counseling process.

While much of the focus of occupational choice is on the major productive role of the individual (i.e., the worker role), occupational choice is a process involving many decisions about life roles. For example, becoming a volunteer, pursuing an amateur activity, preparing for retirement, and deciding how to replace the homemaker role when children leave home are examples of situations requiring an occupational choice. Therapists can bring the same issues and procedures to these choices as to the choice of the worker role. Additionally, they can enable people to identify what needs are met in other continuing or future roles so as to clarify the main purposes of these occupational choices.

Leisure Counseling. The occupational therapist's role as a leisure counselor extends from concern for people's temporal adaptation and their ability to find meaning in play or leisure. The occupational therapist views leisure as one role within the total occupational life-style of the individual. In leisure counseling, the therapist engages in a collaborative problem-solving endeavor with the goal of enhancing the client's ability to independently plan and use leisure time. The process is more involved than simply exploring or enacting leisure interests—it entails identification of the client's values as they pertain to both work and play and of the client's current and anticipated roles and determination of the presence or absence of skills that will support a leisure role.

Occupational therapists encounter many clients for whom leisure counseling is appropriate. Workaholics, socially isolated individuals such as a mother of five children or a previous drug abuser, or a retiree may be potential candidates.[46] A leisure counseling program can also be part of a transitional discharge planning program for psychiatric patients.

A counseling continuum exists for the development of leisure behavior.[46] In this continuum, optimal leisure behavior is self-chosen and independently enacted; that is, the leisure activity is chosen for its own sake, and the client is intrinsically motivated. At the other end of the spectrum is leisure behavior that is dependent and determined by therapy. In other words, the client does not have the skills or resources to actively and independently pursue leisure, but must learn these skills in the context of therapy.

Kolodner[79] describes a transitional program that meets the needs of clients who fall somewhere between these two ends. The program begins with an initial interview in which the interest checklist is used to help the client ascertain interests and skills. Following this session, the therapist investigates community possibilities for enacting at least two of the client's expressed interests. In a future meeting, the therapist gives the client such information as names of agencies or programs, fees, times and dates for activities, and locations. From this information, a program is selected, and plans are made for the client to attend a session. If the client is hesitant about making the initial contact, either another client or the therapist accompanies the person to the activity. After the client's first attendance at the activity, the therapist and client meet again to evaluate the experience. Thus, the client moves from structure and support to gradual independent leisure in the community.

The following is an example of a leisure planning unit for hospitalized psychiatric patients at an earlier stage of leisure behavior. Referrals to this group were based on an inability to identify interests, poor use of free time in the hospital, difficulty scheduling time, and a lack of awareness of community resources or of how to find out about things to do. Group activities began with an examination of how patients' time was presently structured by the hospital program and how they would ideally like to structure their time after discharge. The next sessions were devoted to values clarification activities in which patients identified activities they enjoyed and characteristics of these activities (such as whether or not they were social, expensive, and so on). To help identify new interests, hobby and sports books were brought to group meetings, and patients were asked to choose an activity from these books to carry out on the ward during the week. The next major activity was typically an outing to the local library, where group members collected information on current community events and planned, in pairs, three possible Saturday outings, one of which would be carried out before the next group meeting. When the group reconvened members reported on their trips and then planned a final activity that would be engaged in by the whole group in the last session. This was a time-limited group that moved from ward uses of free time to planning group and community leisure activities.

Cantor[18] describes preretirement planning for individuals who, because of the changes introduced by retirement, may be unable to reorganize or re-balance their use of time. This program begins with clients completing an

100

activities configuration, to identify their current balance of work, play, and self-care, as well as the source of motivation for these activities, and a self-evaluation of how well they perform them. In the second stage of counseling, the client develops a profile of personal time use and then determines areas to change or maintain. The third stage is a search for alternatives, adaptations, or rearrangements leading to the eventual selection of new options for the client's use of time.

Leisure counseling thus draws on the occupational therapist's skills in helping individuals to define their needs, interests, and ability to satisfy these needs and interests, and to locate community resources where leisure interests can be pursued.[46]

The Therapeutic Use of Self in Occupational Therapy

The importance of the self as a therapeutic agent is a general theme in the training of most mental health workers. It implies that the therapist's personal attributes, actions, and reactions are an essential component of therapy.

The goal of the classical psychoanalytic relationship was to achieve an emotional bond between the therapist and the patient that would result in the unfolding of a series of psychodynamics. The patient would project feelings onto this new relationship and recreate earlier relationships from his or her childhood. The therapist was largely passive and commented only rarely, offering interpretations when he or she felt the patient was "ready" to accept them. Neo-Freudians objected to the classical view of the therapist as a tabula rasa, or blank sheet, upon which the patient replayed the drama of childhood relationships. They argued that the therapist's own behaviors contributed as much to the patient's actions as did such psychodynamic processes as transference. Humanists and existentialists went even further, suggesting that the classical model gave the therapist too much importance and control over the relationship because the therapist ultimately and noncollaboratively set treatment goals for the patient. They advocated a nondirective role for the therapist with the patient being responsible for decisions about his or her life.

The humanistic or client-centered approach to therapy has had a pervasive impact on mental health professionals, including occupational therapists.[45] Dunning[31] described the application of humanism to the role of the occupational therapist, stressing that therapists engage in an "authentic" relationship with their clients, accepting the clients' goals and not imposing their own. In building and consolidating this relationship, activity became "a bridge for the relationship to travel on" (p. 475).[31] This notion of the activity as a bridge, however, represents a crucial dilemma to understanding the therapeutic relationship in occupational therapy. If activity is viewed only as a means to some other end, then the value of occupation as a worthwhile human endeavor is denigrated.

What is required to appreciate the therapeutic use of self in occupational therapy is the recognition that human relations include many types of bonds, mutual expectancies, and responses. The classic therapeutic relationship, with its focus on feelings and unconscious elements in the relationship, is only one of many important ways in which human beings relate to each other. In humans, another entire domain of relations can be recognized, those related to productivity and to recreation, festivity, and ritual. These relationships belong to the general class of occupation and are the relationships associated with work and play. The therapeutic use of self in occupational therapy derives its nature from the genre and ethos of these relationships; thus, when engaging clients in occupations, the therapist assumes the role of teacher, supervisor, coach, player, craftsperson, and so forth. Each of these roles contributes to a therapeutic use of self unique to occupational therapy.

Two sets of relationships characterize the use of self in occupational therapy. One set of relations emerges from the therapist's classic function of engaging patients and clients in productive occupations. When a therapist seeks to induce a person to engage in an art, craft, or other productive occupation, he or she must instruct, coach, and supervise, provide support and encouragement, be a role model, and so on. As is obvious from these behaviors, the therapist's function centers on the patient's performance in the occupation and derives its purpose from their joint efforts to engage in a productive enterprise. In the role of instructor, the therapist becomes someone who must know how to do the activity, who values the occupation enough to want to share this knowledge, and who is able to accept the learner's own motives and values pertaining to the occupation and the process of learning. Also, as an instructor, the therapist must be able to diagnose a person's strengths and weaknesses and the constraints and resources in the environment that will affect learning.

When the therapist serves as a role model, he or she communicates that the endeavor is one that requires correct knowledge of procedure, application of personal energy, perseverance, and willingness of the learner to imitate and take advice from the more knowledgeable person. These communications about the reality of productive enterprise are often those that psychosocially dysfunctional people have not had access to in the course of their life experiences.

Related to such task performance, the therapist often serves as a source of hope to the patient, pointing out the worth of struggle by enumerating the possibilities and criteria of success. The therapist is also an important source of affirmation of success and must honestly praise and rejoice in the success of clients. In the context of productive occupation, the therapeutic interaction is built around enabling people to acquire the emotional and informational resources they need to enter a productive role. An apprentice-like association between therapist and client is the key to this therapeutic relationship.[17]

A second major set of behaviors related to the therapeutic use of self in occupational therapy pertains to the play occupations used as therapy. In play, the goal of participants is the expression of common values; affirmation of common humanity and common circumstance; the discovery of new modes of being and experiencing; the celebration of existence, accomplishment, and survival of hardship; the relief from the efforts of labor; and similar emotions and thoughts. All participants in festivity, celebration, playful competition, and other forms of human play come to a common ground and participate in parallel relationships. Hence, the therapist assumes a commonality with all the players and participates genuinely with them in playing. The therapist must be truly participating or else the spirit and ethos of the activity will not emerge and invite participation.

Certain functions are common to both the productive and playful sets of relationships. The first is that the therapist is consistently a creator of meaning. She or he does this by establishing an external order or dramatic context, within which certain behaviors are expected or relevant and others are out of context or irrelevant.[4,120] Meaning is also created when the therapist believes in the value of the activity and cares deeply about the modality itself.[4] Finally the therapist's ability to understand and manage the environment allows him or her to manipulate the setting to contribute to the creation of meaning.

The second function is that of systems analyst. The therapist becomes a creative problem solver, a hypothesis tester, and a provider of feedback.[57] Finally, the therapist becomes both an advocate for clients, enabling them to locate community resources, and a modulator of the environment, seeking to adjust its demands to match the client's potential for action.[134]

The implications of these modes of therapeutic use of self in occupational therapy is that the therapist must be an expert in the nature of occupations, their requirements, their moods, and their pertinent human relations. Similarly, the therapist must be an expert in analyzing the social and physical contexts for occupations and in identifying both individual and environmental resources and constraints for productive behavior. Without an appreciation of the modes of existence and coexistence represented in the occupational efforts of humans, the occupational therapist cannot make effective therapeutic use of self in the manner that is unique to and important for occupational therapy. This principle was stated very simply in the early literature of the field when writers often noted that the therapist must be a craftsperson and a sportsperson, must have an appreciation of music and dance, and must value the occupations used as therapy for their own sake, for their worthiness to solicit human participation.

The Use of Occupations as Therapy

The oldest and most central role of occupational therapists is that of directly engaging people in occupations as treatment. The history of occupational therapy reveals that a broad spectrum of activities have been considered under the rubric of occupation and used for therapy.[67] The earliest and continuing conceptualization of occupation is that it consists of those behaviors with which people fill the majority of their time. Broadly speaking, all forms of work, play, and self-care are types of occupations.

In the early years of this century, many types of play activities were used. These included art, dance, music, theater and drama, and games and sports. The emphasis of the early leaders of occupational therapy on the playful and creative side of human nature and its role in facilitating healthy adaptation supported this wide use of play activities. However, changes occurred as therapists became embarrassed with their "play lady" image and tended to move away from many playful forms of therapy. Arts and crafts were retained apparently because they had an element of productivity and because they simulated work.

Perhaps the occupation most consistently of concern to psychosocial occupational therapists was self-care. Slagle's early programs of habit training focused on this aspect of occupation, and therapists have continued to develop and use training programs for improved self-care of people with psychosocial dysfunction.

At this point in the history of the field, one might properly ask what occupations are suitable for occupational therapy. The response should come from an examination of what constitutes the occupational behaviors that are currently part of the culture. The changing and varied occupational forms that manifest themselves in the everyday life of society should determine what is useful for therapy. Should arts and crafts lose their place in modern society, their relevance to occupational therapy would diminish. If other behaviors emerge as a form of major occupation (for example, computer based activities), then they should find their way into occupational therapy clinics and programs. The field must be attuned to the occupational life of the culture and adjust its therapeutic media accordingly.

Because many subcultures exist in the United States, occupational therapists must be prepared to offer a wide range of occupations as therapy. What is meaningful to a New York theater director will probably not interest a midwestern farmer. The life occupations of a ghetto youth will differ from the interests and abilities of an elderly middle class lawyer. The common denominator among these people is that they have a human urge to explore and master their worlds, which manifests itself in ways relevant to their socio-cultural environments. To be truly effective, occupational therapists must be prepared to offer this range of occupations. Consequently, the following sections describe a wide range of occupations (dance, arts and crafts, games, play, sport, music, theater, work) as the media of occupational therapy. The most central issue for occupational therapy is the art and science which is the basis for using various media as therapy.[132] Thus, this section begins with a perspective on the art and science of using occupation as a health determinant.

The Art and Science of Occupational Therapy Media. A past approach to psychosocial occupational therapy was the use of media as tools of a psychoanalytic therapy. That is, activities were used as arenas in which patients unconsciously revealed and released feelings through the characteristics of their performances. Thus, therapists designed assessment batteries in which patients created collages, clay objects, and fingerpaintings that were then interpreted by therapists for their symbolic and feeling themes.[2,15,82,83] In parallel fashion, the media were used as cathartic mechanisms whereby patients could express and release pent-up feelings. One hammered out anger, portrayed loneliness in blue watercolors, and enacted a need for affection in psychodrama. Even more classical Freudian approaches were used to help patients gratify immature or blocked needs. Thus, anal fixations were worked out in clay, oral gratification was received through a cooking group, and so on.[35]

This approach to occupational therapy in psychosocial practice is best left to the category of historical curiosity for several reasons. First, it is becoming more recognized that psychoanalytic approaches are best used with the patient who is articulate and who can afford the luxury of a longstanding analytic relationship; however, occupational therapists must be willing to relate methods to patients' needs and problems. The patient population seen by occupational therapists in psychosocial practice is more often the chronic patient whose competence is highly questionable. The majority of these patients suffer primarily from an inability to occupy themselves in a productive and self-satisfying manner. They lack the skills for action, the habits for an organized life-style, and the roles that give them identity and make them acceptable to society. Further, those who have been competent and who now suffer from emotional disturbance often do so from a failure to find meaning in their lives, and the problem is one of bringing their values, goals, and personal view of self into focus and relating them to activity in the real world.

Another reason for giving up the psychoanalytic approach is that occupational therapy should serve as a socializing environment in which patients learn how to construct and organize their actions and identities. This particular orientation is largely incompatible with either an exclusively analytic or combined analytic/competency approach. Reasons for this are found in the communications given when occupations are used as therapy and the context of their presentation to patients. One of the most basic lessons of life is that there is a time and place for everything. Patients in psychiatric care are often heavily engaged in the business of working through pathological or painful feeling states. A great deal of attention is paid to the experience and expression of painful emotions. When such an orientation pervades much of the patient's life, it becomes difficult to discriminate when and where healthy expression of negative feelings should occur.

Of all therapies, occupational therapy should have the most fundamental commitment to the process of doing and to there being a time and a place for performance where negative feelings are tolerated and controlled while the person works toward the positive feelings of accomplishment, satisfaction, control, and self-worth.[37] Such feeling states as anger and self-satisfaction are notoriously incompatible. The importance of occupational therapy as a very special area within the psychosocial treatment arena—one which demands performance and which duly rewards it with recognition—must not be underestimated. The fundamental message of occupational therapy is that positive feelings accrue through the risk-taking, the creativity, and the effort of engaging in work and play. That message should come through clearly in occupational therapy.

Additionally, one should give serious consideration to the possibility that an eclectic approach combining the competency orientation and the expression of unconscious feelings may bear an inherently inconsistent and highly confusing message, because of its potential double-bind communication. In competency-oriented practice, the patient derives satisfaction and feelings of self-worth through completion of some performance or some product that he or she has planned, chosen, and executed. Here the message is that conscious, willful application of effort yielded some worthy outcome. The analytic approach, which views activity as the product or expression of unconscious feeling otherwise not accessible, offers a contradictory message. It suggests the product of performance is shaped by unconscious and negative forces. It appears inconsistent and self-contradictory that a hammered ashtray should be at once an expression of ability and effort as well as the manifestation of latent anger, or that a painting should express insecurity while being an example of competent execution of technique and aesthetic. For patients who are struggling for evidence of their worth and ability, the suggestion that unconscious forces move and direct performances runs too high a risk of undermining a sense of accomplishment or providing conflicting versions of performance. It would do little for one's feelings of competence to be confused about whether the choice of the color red was a manifestation of one's ability to artfully produce or of one's anger.

The fundamental occupational therapy hypothesis is that people can become competent and confident through what they do. Doing enables people to become more fully human as they develop their potential and earn their membership in the culture through their contributions. Operationalization of that hypothesis is a complex enterprise requiring the effort and attention of the field. Dispersing the field's efforts to multiple orientations and techniques does little to fulfill this mandate.

The art and science of occupational therapy underlying the therapeutic use of occupations is based in the understanding of the health-giving nature of occupation and the cultural and personal significance of occupation. As the culture develops and changes or varies among different groups, media will necessarily change and vary. Whereas looms filled the clinics in past generations, computers will likely be important in the future as therapeutic media.[54] For one patient in one part of the country, music may mean a simple hand-wrought instrument, while for another, it is appreciation of the classics. For some people manual labor is demeaning, while for others it signifies the reason and worth of their existence. Recognition of these differences and the flexibility to use a wide range of media as part of the art and science of occupational therapy practice are essential.

Play. The play of childhood is a singularly important contributor to competence in adulthood.[111] Occupational therapists have long acknowledged play to be a critical developmental phenomenon that facilitates adaptation toward adult occupational behavior. In play, children learn symbols or rules that serve as internal maps for acting on the world.[111,113] Play is an important learning medium because it involves the use of musculoskeletal, neurological, and symbolic components of skill;[40] because it incorporates an attitude of curiosity and a state of optimal neurological excitation or arousal;[40,86,113,126] and because it provides a safe context for experimentation. Play facilitates and mirrors the developmental process.[40,125] Early play facilitates sensorimotor development and simple social interaction skills. Later, it develops more complex social behaviors, mastery over tool use, and assumption of roles.

The approaches to using play as therapy are multiple and often complex. To elicit play the environment must have sufficient and suitable objects and people, there should be novelty and opportunities for exploration, repetition, and imitation.[26,40] The approach to eliciting play through environmental manipulation thus includes the use of objects, people, and events. Play activities must also be chosen for the appropriate developmental level of children.

Florey[40] and Michelman[97] offer excellent schemas for identifying the appropriate objects, people, and procedures at different levels of play.

The major rationale underlying the use of play as a therapeutic medium is the identification of skill deficits that can be attributed to a lack or paucity of play experiences. Robinson[113] provides a series of questions to be used to guide judgments about whether a child plays and how well he or she plays. The play history interview also provides data on the quality and quantity of play experiences. Following the identification of children's play deficits, therapists can determine the type of play that would facilitate the development and acquisition of skills. Play is an appropriate arena in which to affect change in all three constituents of skills, because it is a holistic phenomenon.

Games. A subclass of play, games are motivating because they reduce the severity of consequences while still allowing the individual to employ his or her abilities and take risks in situations of competition, uncertainty, and chance. The advent of simulated games has paved the way for a new understanding of gaming technique as a means of encapsulating some complex aspect of reality and allowing one to compete, solve problems, pursue strategies, and receive realistic feedback on consequences.[111]

In adolescent and childhood psychosocial treatment settings, games are routinely used as forms of normal recreation. Here their therapeutic properties are seen largely in the context of providing normal patterns of childhood and adolescent behavior to occupy patients' time. However, games have been used in more specific ways in occupational therapy. For example, Carey[19] explored the utility of games in developing an appreciation of the nature of rules and the reciprocal behavior of following rules in juvenile delinquent youths. According to research and clinical observation, juvenile delinquents exhibit less ability to engage in and enjoy competitive game situations. The program was thus designed to enable delinquent youths to develop a sense of rules through competitive play. A series of game-playing sessions were followed by discussions of what happens when rules are broken, why rules are followed, how rules allow people to play the game together, the implications of cheating, and the nature of competition, winning, and losing.

Hurff[56] created several table games and adapted commercial games to simulate real life situations. These enabled people to try out problem-solving approaches and strategies for social interaction and to learn some concrete skills. This program of games was devised for developmentally disabled adolescents and adults; the program appears to be easily generalizable to all populations of psychosocially disabled people who are experiencing difficulty in daily living skills and judgments. Hurff provides a useful overview of the literature on games as learning situations and a helpful list of properties of games that facilitate the development of skills. These can be used as guidelines for selecting or constructing games.

Hurff observed that her program of games provided patients with the opportunity to experience a variety of simulated situations that arise in community life. One particularly interesting aspect of the games was the simulation of emergency situations. Allowing people to experience and respond to these circumstances in the game facilitated their adaptive response when such situations arose in real life. Overall, simulated games appear to be useful preludes to actual community training and experience.

Sports. Sports are a natural part of everyday life. Many Americans recreate as sport spectators and participants. In early occupational therapy, sports were valued for their ability to teach participants a sense of sportsmanship, which was viewed as an antecedent to citizenship or participation in everyday social reality.[67]

While the use of sports in occupational therapy has been less widespread in recent years, they remain a potentially rich medium for therapeutic application for several reasons. First, their widespread popularity makes them attractive to many people. Second, sports are highly variable and adaptable. They can range from such simple procedures as tag to complex games with many rules and players, such as baseball and basketball. They can be solitary activities such as swimming, fishing, or running, or group activities with highly organized interrelationships. They can involve very simple gross motor movements or quite demanding feats of coordination. The advent of new games[42,43] that have been incorporated into many occupational therapy programs has allowed a creative and noncompetitive use of sporting activities.

While sports have a wide variety of potentially therapeutic properties, three are notable. First, the excitement of competition and/or cooperation tends to attract people, often eliciting performance not otherwise possible.

The second property of sports is their unique ability to teach people role behavior.[69,126] In sports, people assume a variety of roles and have the opportunity to understand how roles determine one's contribution to the team or group and how roles guide reciprocal behavior between participants.

Finally, sports, both in participatory and spectator forms, generate enthusiasm and a sense of belonging to social groups.[126] Everything from the homecoming game to the World Series has a special way of bringing individuals a sense of community and common purpose. No doubt, society needs its games to keep members feeling that they are part of the whole. Games can help overcome feelings of alienation and solidify one's attempts to be a part of a group.

King[72] developed an approach to using sporting activities based on concepts of neurological function and dysfunction in some psychiatric patients. While her primary aim in using games and sports was to facilitate sensory integration, she recognized the importance of mind-body interactions and, thus, the necessity of incorporating desired sensory and motor experiences into sport-like activities. Recognizing that neurological changes could be elicited only when proper mental and conscious experiences are involved, she incorporated "elements of skill, chance surprise, incongruity, and suspense" (p. 535)[72] in the activities in order to make them attractive and meaningful, and to elicit a sense of pleasurable participation on behalf of patients. King's approach is an example of the hierarchical principle that when one wishes to correct a deficit in one constitutent of skill, other constituents and their relationships must be recognized.

Kaplan[58] developed a group for low level psychiatric patients of all diagnoses. Her goal was to provide simple adaptations of sports with low demands for both rules and behavior. One example of her adapted sports is a game in which people throw a Nurf ball to other seated members in a circle, while engaging in a parallel verbal behavior such as naming the person to whom the ball is thrown or naming a member of some class of objects (e.g., a type of car) without repeating anything another person has already said. She also employs an adapted form of soccer involving kicking a ball from seated positions and attempting to get it past another person's chair. Kaplan's procedure incorporates simple rules, skills, and roles into an activity that has an element of fun and moderate competition along with cooperation and reality-orientation. The games elicit participation from patients who do not participate in verbal groups or other activities.

Kielhofner and Miyake[69] used sports with mentally retarded adults to elicit a variety of motor, psychosocial, and social behavior changes. These people were unaccustomed to the movements, attitudes, and rules and behaviors of the sport activities. Therapists participated in the sports as peers and as coaches, keeping up the mood and continuity of the game. Over a period of time the program progressed from simple sports such as games of tag to football, frisbee, and baseball, complex games with multiple roles and teams.

Performing Arts. The performing arts include such occupations as drama, dance, film and video, music, magic, puppetry, storytelling, and mime. Many of these media hold a less prominent place in occupational therapy today than in the past. However, their substantial possibilities for therapeutic application are being increasingly recognized. One important reason for the inclusion of such occupations in psychosocial practice is the need for a wide range of media to suit the particular tastes and values of different persons. Not all people are oriented to or find meaning in creative arts that result in the production of an object. They may prefer those that have public performance as their goal. Performing arts also provide opportunities for different kinds of action, emotion, and cognition—as well as a very different social organization—than do creative arts.

Music and drama, for instance, are important agents of socialization in many societies and subcultures. For adolescents, being familiar with the prevailing musical hits and knowing the current dance steps are essential parts of fitting in with one's peers. For certain adults, church singing and piano singalongs are favorite forms of recreation. Drama is closely linked to ritual and in some societies is a means of passing along the traditions and history of the group. In addition, the prescribed role relationships that may exist in drama, folk dancing, music ensembles, and so on provide opportunities to learn and practice different roles in the context of highly coordinated and cooperative behavior. Thus, the expressive arts offer a variety of opportunities for people to learn and practice skills, develop social interaction and role behavior, deepen their appreciation of the cultural meanings of their environments, and experience the success that accrues from personal and mutual application of human effort. Finally, the public nature of expressive arts provides via the intended and actual audience a point of reference and a source of feedback that facilitates self-assessment.

Goldstein and Collins[47] note an additional advantage of film and video as permanent performing media, since they "require integration into the user's environment; that is, one needs to be in a specific environment to take a picture of that environment" (p. 530).[47] They describe a videotape project with hospitalized adolescents that capitalized on the cultural relevance of television to this age group. This project enabled the teenagers to learn how to use equipment, to assume different production roles and levels of responsibility, to achieve some control over their experiences of hospitalization, and to explore issues pertaining to health care and illness in the scripts.

Performing arts also provide opportunities for individuals to recognize, affirm, and appreciate the significant events of a culture. For instance, a Christmas play and talent show allows participants to explore and express the meanings of the holiday. The collective efforts required to execute a play, a circus, a variety show, a musical, or a dance presentation have an unusual organizing effect on patients. Typically, people who have seemed incompetent or withdrawn suddenly muster the ability to perform and maintain a protracted contact with the reality of some purposeful action in the world. The ambience of the performing arts and the way in which they signify the connection between performer and society make them immediately useful as a means of bringing people into the reality of social life. Further, their role as carriers of emotional and symbolic messages such as beauty, hope, courage, joy, triumph over suffering, and so forth makes them especially appropriate as experiences that teach values and meaning to participants.

Arts and Crafts. For a period of time, the utility of arts and crafts in occupational therapy was questioned, in part due to the general devaluation of "handmade" objects in American culture as brought on by mass production and consumerism. Today, there is a resurrection of handcraft represented not only in the increasing number of people engaging in crafts, but in the increased commercial value of handmade items.

Perhaps the single most imporant contribution to the field's understanding of the value of arts and crafts was made by Reilly[109] in her statement that "man, through the use of his hands as they are energized by mind and will, can influence the state of his own health" (p. 2). Though she did not intend the statement to be solely on behalf of the arts and crafts, it served as a reaffirmation of their importance as a therapeutic tool, since crafts bind thought and action. One can view art and craft as a subcategory of play that embodies its freedom, joy, and creativity while resulting in a tangible, useful, and aesthetic object. Thus, while craft is playfully done, it can serve a productive end. As such, it is an important bridge between play and work.

Crafts embody a value system (standards of performance and utility) and procedural rules that make them organizing activities. To engage in the craft, one must correctly apply the rules. One is energized by the possibility of excellence in the craft and the potential for beauty and utility in the product. Crafts can be important simulators of work satisfaction and work conditions.[23]

Crafts lend themselves to both individual and cooperative group processes. The therapist often serves as a kind of master craftsperson who must select tools and materials and demonstrate techniques, serving as an inspiration and a role model to participants. Crafts can be integrated into actual life situations when persons make objects to decorate or to function within their own living spaces or as gifts. Art and craft organized into the individual's life are more meaningful.

A number of therapeutic properties of arts and crafts have been identified.[23,109] They include opportunities for problem solving; learning to deal with materials and people in productive situations; the ability to develop a positive self-image and increased confidence from accomplishment; the potential to productively contribute to society; the development of skills that can carry over into one's life-style; and orientation to the reality of work.

Work. The value of work as therapy has long been recognized, beginning with the efforts of moral treatment practitioners. Occupational therapists have continued to use various forms of work as a part of their therapeutic programs.

Noting that hospitalization often resulted in atrophy of work skills and work roles, Reilly[110] argued that work should be incorporated into all adult therapeutic programs. She also pointed out that for the adult, work is a necessary component of the balance of occupation in daily life. One cannot have true leisure unless it has been earned through work.

Forms of work that are used in therapy vary greatly both in content and in organization. Work may simply be the completion of simple chores on the ward or completion of clerical tasks in a work module organized in occupational therapy. On the other hand, it may involve more serious volunteer work in the institution or the community or even reimbursed labor under the auspices of job training programs. Generally, more serious forms of work are seen as the final phase in a continuum of treatment for people with psychosocial dysfunction. Work is the most demanding of life tasks; it tends to be public, often involves drudgery, and requires substantial ability, commitment, and perseverance.

One approach to providing work for patients with psychosocial problems is to organize simple work modules within the occupational therapy workshop or clinic. In one work program, adolescent inpatients performed different tasks pursuant to making a large table game for the ward. Jobs were posted on the ward, and patients applied and were interviewed by a volunteer who also served as job supervisor. Patients were "hired" for the program to perform such jobs as carpenter, painter, and janitor. Hours were assigned, and patients punched in and out of work. They were paid in the form of tokens that could be used to purchase food and other objects.

Another way that meaningful work roles have been incorporated into a treatment program can be seen in community mental health programs for long-term treatment of psychiatric clients. In a clubhouse program based on Fountain House, members filled needed and important roles related to clubhouse maintenance. They performed jobs such as the clerical tasks of writing, artwork, production, and distribution of member newspapers; food preparation and the associated tasks of menu-planning, money management, serving, and cleanup; and tasks related to special events throughout the year. In addition to these tasks, members were responsible for orienting, touring, and being "buddies" to new members. All jobs were selected for their necessity in developing and maintaining the clubhouse and for their similarity to normal everyday responsibilities and activities. Occasional work projects based on subcontracting from other agencies were also accepted and performed by some members for wages. Finally, volunteer opportunities were made available to interested members. The clubhouse operation depended on the productive participation of its members. Both the maintenance of the organization itself and the services it offered to members and to the community relied on the efforts of members. There were opportunities for members to engage in meaningful work tasks with identifiable purposes, to collaborate with each other, and to contribute toward the maintenance of an organization to which they belonged. The organization of work into a program such as this is probably the most relevant kind of experience that adults with psychosocial dysfunction can have. It serves as a bridge between earlier states of disorganization and the organized labor required for productive community life. However, it does so in the context of a real and functioning institution.

Goodwin[48] describes another, often used approach of placing patients in jobs within the institution. This was once a major function of occupational therapy and was referred to as industrial therapy. The occupational therapist identified supervisors, who then either used patients as volunteers or reimbursed them for work within their departments. The occupational therapist was involved at both ends—consulting with the supervisors and counseling and performing training and mutual problem solving with the person placed on the job.

Another approach is the placement of people in industry in the community. DeMars[25] describes such a program in which she arranged with local industry for retarded people to be placed as janitors in actual job situations. A final level of involvement of the occupational therapist has been in the sheltered workshop. Such programs generally provide reimbursed work that is subcontracted from various groups. Therapists in such settings function in roles from job supervisor and work simplification expert to overall manager of the workshop.

Activities of Daily Living (ADL). Historically, occupational therapists have been concerned with activities of daily living as both a set of skills to be learned or maintained and as providing activities that place demands on clients for normal behavior while in treatment. ADL skills are necessary for adaptive, independent functioning and they reflect the client's self-image. Many of these activities could be considered as hobbies or as work if performed with different intent. Mosey[101] describes ADL as referring to "all those activities one must engage in or accomplish to be able to participate with comfort in other facets of life" (p. 75). The list of ADL areas of concern to occupational therapy includes the following: grooming; personal hygiene; food preparation, shopping, and nutrition; general home maintenance; communications, such as writing notes and using the telephone; money management; ability to arrange for transportation; and time management. The need for and nature of competence in each area varies with the individual's life experiences and the requirements of the setting in which the person lives.[71]

ADL programs have continued as a component of many psychosocial occupational therapy programs, whether in acute or chronic care hospitals, in community day treatment programs, or in transitional programs between the hospital and community. In acute care, the goal is usually to maintain the level of functioning rather than to teach new skills.[21] Community treatment programs frequently have ADL skill training components such as job-seeking skills, cooking, and grooming.[14] A lecture approach has also been used by some therapists to teach the ADL skills of homemaking, cooking, and dress-making, among other topics.[24,59] Yet another approach to increasing independence in the area of ADL is illustrated by a "quarterway house" program developed at a state hospital for a group of predischarge patients.[92] They were given increased responsibility for ADL, and the program included task group meetings in which training in areas of cooking, laundering, transportation, money management, shopping, and medications management were covered.

The benefits of ADL training may extend beyond the immediate skills learned. For instance, an intensive community reorientation training in ADL and leisure skills resulted not only in skill learning, but also in greater social interest among group members, increased social competence, and decreased symptomatology.[88]

The Use of Task-Oriented Groups

Groups have been used in occupational therapy throughout its history in a variety of ways. Although there is an extensive body of knowledge on group dynamics and group processes, the types and structures of groups in occupational therapy should reflect both the profession's unique emphasis on the value of occupation and a client/therapist relationship that directly promotes action and competence. Because the field is concerned with occupational groups, understanding of group process should derive from a sociological, as opposed to a psychodynamic, perspective on groups. In practical terms, this translates into asking, for example, how individuals learn and assume various occupational roles in a group, rather than asking how someone uses the group for multiple transference.

Examples of occupational groups found in everyday life include community task forces, political groups, music ensembles, sports teams, clubs, special interest groups such as weight loss groups, work units, parent-teacher groups, and so on. What these groups share is a task orientation—they exist specifically to accomplish some real and substantial activity, such as developing a program policy, winning a game, putting on a performance, or getting a job done. They differ from the type of group usually found in therapeutic settings in that the latter typically emphasize increasing self-understanding, and rely on talking to accomplish this goal. Self-understanding may well be a product of many occupational groups, but it is neither their explicit nor their only intended function.

The use of groups in psychosocial occupational therapy fills several important roles: It provides a recapitulation of productive and playful normal aspects of life; it allows for the development of social behaviors necessary to participating in occupational roles; and it is an arena for the communication of occupational values.

As a socialization process, occupational therapy communicates the expectations of the larger culture. Groups are an intrinsic part of our society, and people naturally belong to or identify with various groups throughout their lives. Donohue,[29] for instance, discusses a group that she labels an identification group. This is a homogeneous age and sex group to which a person naturally belongs. She uses the term "identification" instead of "reference group," because the latter typically implies a choice of wanting to use the group to define oneself. Many psychosocial patients, however, may not aspire toward membership in the reference group assigned to them by society. The identification group can evolve into a true reference group for the patient, however. In the women's identification group described by Donohue, activities included topic-centered discussions of issues such as birth control, child-rearing, and self-defense; experimentation with new behaviors, such as assertiveness and decision making; exercise and aerobics; and a casual coffee and rap session. These are all activities that would conceivably be engaged in by a group of nonhospitalized women meeting socially.

Similarly, Versluys'[127] role-focused groups are designed around the homemaker's role, maintenance of roles enacted by the patient prior to hospitalization, and family roles. The groups enable patients to discover that "they are capable of being productive within their physical and medical limitations" (p. 612) and to remain somewhat involved in the groups to which they belonged in normal life. In the role maintenance group, for instance, group members help one another to find ways in which they can carry out their family, community, and work obligations while they are hospitalized. This has the effects of minimizing the sick role and of helping the patient to maintain control of his or her life.

Occupational therapy literature is replete with examples of groups that have been used to teach daily living skills, social skills, and work skills. Many behaviors that are encompassed by the role of productive participant are best learned in groups. For instance, cooperation, competition, and consensual decision making can all be natural concomitants to various group activities. Fidler[36] describes the task group as "a shared working experience" where "alternate patterns of functioning can be considered and tested" (p. 45). She highlights the value of task groups as focusing on active and current involvement in a situation that closely simulates real life experience and demands for skilled, responsible, interpersonal behavior.

Skill development groups give patients the opportunity to receive feedback from their peers, to serve as role models for one another, and to experiment with new behaviors in a setting where experimentation is the norm. The therapeutic social club, which uses community resources and settings, enables former mental patients to develop leisure and interpersonal skills in a situation that bridges the gap between hospital and community.[30] Heine[53] described a daily living group that provided didactic and experiential learning in such areas as job hunting and interviewing, leisure planning, using the community, and finding living arrangements, among others. Meacham and Lindemann[95] developed a summer program for adolescents organized around work, social, self-care, and academic skill development in group settings. An assembly project gave teenagers the chance to produce salable products in an assembly-line situation, while the luncheon party unit involved members in learning about nutrition, planning and executive meals, and preparing a formal party for invited guests.

Mosey[100] offered guidelines for structuring task groups that would facilitate different levels of interpersonal skills; these groups range from a parallel level of activity, where individuals work on their own projects, to a mature, co-operative level, where members share responsibility for a completion of a major total group product. The importance of these guidelines lies in the knowledge that many work and leisure occupations are not only conducted in group settings but also require cooperative or team efforts. In addition, most occupational roles are learned and carried out in interpersonal contexts,[101,127] and even roles that are eventually done somewhat independently, such as homemaker, are initially learned in a social situation (the family).

One example of how patients can assume both cooperative and individual roles can be found in German's[44] avocational interest group. The specific purpose of this group was to enable patients to develop interests in hobbies that could be pursued outside of the hospital. The group was structured with a short workshop period in which patients moved in and out of teaching and learning roles with one another. In addition, the use of written instructions and catalogues encouraged patients to independently pursue their interests outside the group.

In order to successfully communicate relevant occupational values, the group environment must be structured to be consistent with the demands of the group task. If a goal for therapy is to socialize individuals with little or no work history into a worker role, then a work group must embody, through explicit rules, the norms and values that are associated with work by society at large. If a new member perceives that others in the group consider their work to be important and preparatory for moving on to a job in another setting, then he or she will be inclined to adopt this attitude as well. Along with the attitude, the individual will feel group pressure to come on time, to interact in a manner that is appropriate for a work setting, and so forth. Donohue's[29] identification group operationalized this principle by using activities common to women in their daily lives, as well as an organizational format conducive to these activities. Aerobics sessions recreated the atmosphere of an adult education class, while the rap sessions recalled an informal living room or kitchen gathering. The leader acted as a group member, role model, and guide, helping other members to take on these roles as well. This structure, however, would not suffice for a work-skills group. There the emphasis would be on creating an atmosphere similar to what one would encounter in the real work world. Social and personal conversation would be minimal, and the leader would more appropriately function as supervisor or boss, rather than as group member.

THE OCCUPATIONAL THERAPIST AS ENVIRONMENTAL MANAGER

CREATING A CONTEXT FOR TREATMENT:

Occupational therapy influences the attitudes, conscious processes, and recovery of patients by how it organizes the environment.

Therapist's attitudes and indications about the activity and its value all influence how patients experience therapy.

Therapy ultimately has a role in constructing or reconstructing reality for patients via the messages contained in the therapeutic environment.

The environment of therapy is conceptualized as a context that guides and defines behavior and experiences.

These contexts may include exploration, festivity and ritual, sport, craft, work and play as a value, and an educational milieu.

Contexts are communicated by physical and architectural properties of a setting; dress, behavior, values, and ideas of people in a setting; and verbal and nonverbal communication.

Occupational therapy includes a context of competence by structuring the environment to match people's abilities.

MANAGING THE COMMUNITY ENVIRONMENT:

Occupational therapy has a developing role in managing the community environment; there is potential for occupational therapists to assume leadership positions in community mental health programming.

The community is a natural setting for occupational therapy since it provides a meaningful and normal context for learning skills.

Community work in comparison to the hospital is less structured, without physical boundaries, and has more flexible and complex administrative and co-worker relationships, and a relatively nonmedical orientation.

The community therapist must be familiar with community standards; work with a wide range of people and agencies; have a broader understanding of the life situations, culture, history, and environments of clients; and be able to assume roles as program director and consultant.

Community settings include residential programs, halfway houses, clubhouse programs, day treatment, sheltered workshops, quarterway houses, partial hospitalization, and prevention programs for the well elderly.

Models of community programming in which occupational therapists have been involved include aftercare programs to aid adjustment and promote independence, work-oriented day care programs, the clubhouse model (Fountain House), neighborhood extension of activity therapy, and a preventive activity program for elderly people.

THERAPIST AS CO-PROBLEM SOLVER AND CO-PLANNER

Counseling is within the purview of occupational therapy when it focuses on facilitating a person's participation in a pattern of healthy occupation.

Time management planning and problem solving:
- are based on a framework of temporal adaptation;
- focus on balance in daily life behavior; the match of values, interests, and goals to time use; role balance and performance; and temporal adjustments for pathology;
- aim at establishing a schedule of healthy occupation for clients to follow.

Occupational choice counseling:
- occurs when occupational choice is delayed or when a poor choice has been made;
- aims to having people find and operationalize work, play, and other roles consistent with their abilities and desires.

Leisure counseling:
- extends from a concern for overall temporal adaptation and the need for people to find meaning in play or leisure;
- involves identification of clients' values, roles, and skills to support leisure activities;
- applies to people such as workaholics, socially isolated individuals, or retirees with difficulty adjusting to leisure;

- may be part of a discharge planning or transitional program;
- may be part of a preretirement counseling program.

THE THERAPEUTIC USE OF SELF IN OCCUPATIONAL THERAPY

Concepts of the therapeutic use of self have evolved substantially since they originally grew out of psychoanalytic approaches.

In occupational therapy the therapeutic use of self has undergone shifts in emphasis.

Among a variety of human relationships, occupational therapy uses a special class of relationship related to occupation.

The therapeutic relationship in occupational therapy revolves around:
- interactions for accomplishing productive tasks in which people require emotional and information resources to support the struggle to perform competently;
- interactions for accomplishing forms of play such as ritual, celebration, sport, and recreation.

In the therapeutic relationship the occupational therapist influences the creation of the meaning of activities and supports the process of successful performance or participation in an occupation.

In order to enact the therapeutic use of self, the occupational therapist must have expertise in and value the occupations used as therapy.

THE USE OF OCCUPATIONS AS THERAPY

The central role of occupational therapy is providing occupations in which patients and clients participate.

Occupations refer to the broad spectrum of activities in which people engage as part of their routine use of time and include work, play, and self-care.

Emphasis on different types of occupations as therapy has differed over the history of the field.

The criterion for inclusion of occupations as forms of therapy should be their relevance to the culture at large and to the cultural background of people in therapy.

The art and science of occupational therapy media:
- centers on the process of developing competence for performance of work, play, and self-care activities;
- does not include the process of identifying and expressing unconscious feelings;

- is based on the understanding of the health-giving nature of occupation and on understanding the cultural and personal significance of occupation.

Play:
- contributes to the development of competency;
- serves as a therapeutic modality to increase skill and confidence.

Games:
- are a subclass of play that allow people to take risks in controlled and inconsequential contexts;
- may simulate the problems of everyday life and allow practice of problem-solving;
- are part of normal occupational behavior;
- may facilitate the development of moral behavior through appreciation of the functions of rules and their binding nature.

Sports:
- teach participants a sense of sportsmanship;
- evoke motor activity through their motivating properties;
- allow learning of roles, their functions, and reciprocal role relationships.

Performing arts:
- include dance, drama, film and video, music, magic, puppetry, storytelling, and mime;
- can be important forms of socialization and are linked to ritual;
- have a public nature, which means that they provide a point of reference and a source of feedback.

Arts and crafts:
- are enjoying a resurgence of popularity and worth;
- uniquely bind hands and mind to a productive purpose;
- can be integrated into people's life situations;
- can be individual or group activities;
- result in tangible, aesthetic, and useful products.

Work:
- should be a component of all adult therapeutic programs;
- can vary from chores, to work activities in the hospital, to volunteer activities, to actual work training;
- requires integration into a context that gives the work meaning and purpose.

Activities of daily living:
- are both targets and means of therapy;
- include those activities that support participation in other facets of daily life.

THE USE OF TASK-ORIENTED GROUPS

The use of groups in occupational therapy focuses on occupation (i.e., accomplishing tasks).

Groups:
- allow various occupations to take on a real rather than a simulated character;
- facilitate socialization of members into the attitudes and behaviors reflective of similar groups in the culture;
- facilitate social productive role behavior;
- serve as contexts for teaching skills;
- should be structured according to the ethos of groups that are naturally organized to accomplish tasks.

TERMS AND CONCEPTS

closed system	A system that does not interact with its environment and is not alive (e.g., a machine).
competent	Fulfilling the expectations of others.
context	A psychosocial setting that people recognize and that influences how they experience and behave.
custodialism	The process of containing handicapped people in institutions without offering rehabilitation.
cybernetic process	A process of modifying behavior based on feedback.
deinstitutionalization	The placement of people who were formerly in state hospitals into the community along with efforts to reduce the numbers of people sent to state hospitals in the first place.
demoralization	Loss of interest and commitment to one's way of life; a feeling of meaninglessness and hopelessness.
extrinsic motivation	Motivation whose source is not from within the activity itself. Extrinsically motivated behaviors are those done for some underlying motive (e.g., hunger) or motive external to the activity (e.g., payment or social praise) rather than for the activity itself.
fantasy period	A stage in occupational choice when choices are based solely on perceived pleasure in an occupation.

feedback   The return of information to a system concerning the process and outcomes of its action.

goals   Plans for future accomplishments.

gradation   The principle of gradually increasing the complexity and challenge of occupations used as therapy.

habit deterioration   The breakdown of routines of everyday life manifest in chaotic and disorganized daily behavior.

habits   Internal images that trigger and guide routine performance.

habit training   The name for early occupational therapy programs that incorporated full 24-hour schedules of work, play, rest, and sleep. These programs were aimed at restoring healthy patterns of daily occupational behavior.

habituation   A process of developing routine behavior patterns. This term is used to describe the subsystem in the Model of Human Occupation which regulates routine behavior. It includes habits and roles as part of its structure.

hierarchy   The arrangement of phenomena into levels in which higher ones govern and are constrained by the lower.

intake   The importation of information and energy from the environment.

interests   Dispositions to find certain objects or activities pleasurable.

internalized expectations   Expectations for performance associated with a role that one perceives to pertain to oneself.

internalized role   A role and its expectations which one perceives oneself to hold and which one believes others perceive one to hold.

123

intrinsic motivation	Motivation that emanates from the behavior itself rather than from some extraneous motive. Thus, intrinsically motivated activity is activity done for its own sake and not for some extrinsic reward.
mainstreaming	A policy of placing handicapped people in the types of institutions (e.g., schools) where nonhandicapped people are located.
meaningful activity	Activity which relates to a person's values and interests and which provides a sense of accomplishment and worth when it is performed.
normalization	An ideology that believes in giving handicapped people access to resources and circumstances to which the average (normal) member of the community has access.
occupational behavior	The performace of daily work, play, and self-care tasks.
occupational performance	See *occupational behavior*.
occupations	Activities motivated by the urge to explore and master. They generally include work, play, and activities of daily living.
output	The performance of some action by a system.
perceived role incumbance	The belief that one has the status and obligations of a given role and that others perceive likewise.
personal causation	Images one holds concerning one's effectiveness as an actor in the world.
press	The demands of the environment for certain types of behavior.
realistic period	A stage in occupational choice when the person has made a selection and has begun to operationalize the choice through receiving training and so forth.
role	A recognized position or status in a social group which had defined obligation for performance.

role balance   The healthy integration of roles into a routine of behavior satisfying to self and relevant others.

role dysfunction   Imbalance of roles and/or ability to perform the tasks associated with a role or roles.

sense of efficacy A feeling that one is able to competently perform necessary and valued tasks.

socialization   The developmental process of acquiring the attitudes, values, and behavioral norms of a particular social group.

temporal adaptation The organization of daily life behaviors into a satisfying and competent pattern of performance.

tension reduction The release of pent-up psychic energy.

tentative period   A stage in occupational choice when a person has begun to seriously select an occupation based on interests, values, and an understanding of personal capacity.

throughput   The transformation of energy and information within a system and its incorporation into the function and structure of the system. Throughput often results in a change in the structure of a system.

values   Personal images of what is good, right, or otherwise highly desirable.

volition   The process of willing or choosing. The term is used to describe a subsystem in the Model of Human Occupation which is responsible for making choices. According to this theory, volition begins with the urge to explore and master and incorporates one's personal causation, values, and interests.

REFERENCES

1. Ayres, J. *Sensory integration and learning disorders.* Los Angeles: Western Psychological Services, 1972.
2. Azima, H., & Azima, F. J. Outline of a dynamic theory of occupational therapy. *American Journal of Occupational Therapy*, 1959, *13*, 215–221.
3. Barris, R. Environmental interactions: An extension of the model of

human occupation. *American Journal of Occupational Therapy*, 1982, *36*, 637–644.

4. Bateson, G. Communication in occupational therapy. *American Journal of Occupational Therapy*, 1956, *10*, 188.

5. Beard, H. G., Propst, R. N., & Malamud, T. J. The Fountain House model of psychiatric rehabilitation. *Psychosocial Rehabilitation Journal*, 1982, *5*, 47–53.

6. Behnke, C. J. *Examining reliability of the play history*. Unpublished master's project, Department of Occupational Therapy, Virginia Commonwealth University, 1982.

7. Black, M. Adolescent role assessment. *American Journal of Occupational Therapy*, 1976, *30*, 73–79.

8. Bledsoe, N., & Shepherd, J. The preschool play scale. *American Journal of Occupational Therapy*, 1983, in press.

9. Bloomer, J., & Williams, S. The Bay Area Functional Performance Evaluation. In B. Hemphill (Ed.), *The evaluative process in psychiatric occupational therapy*. Thoroughfare, N.J.: Charles B. Slack, 1982.

10. Bockoven, J. S. Challenge of the new clinical approaches. *American Journal of Occupational Therapy*, 1968, *22*, 23–25.

11. Bockoven, J. S. *Moral treatment in community mental health*. New York: Springer Publishing, 1972.

12. Borys, S. Implications of interest theory for occupational therapy. *American Journal of Occupational Therapy*, 1974, *28*, 35–38.

13. Brayman, S. J., Kirby, T. F., Misenheimer, A. M., & Short, M. J. Comprehensive occupational therapy evaluation scale. *American Journal of Occupational Therapy*, 1976, *30*, 94–100.

14. Broekema, M. C., Danz, K. H., & Schloemer, C. U. Occupational therapy in a community aftercare program. *American Journal of Occupational Therapy*, 1975, *29*, 22–27.

15. Buck, R. E., & Provancher, M. A. Magazine picture collages as an evaluative technique. *American Journal of Occupational Therapy*, 1972, *26*, 36–39.

16. Burke, J. P. A clinical perspective on motivation: Pawn versus origin. *American Journal of Occupational Therapy*, 1977, *31*, 254–258.

17. Burke, J. P., Miyake, S., Kielhofner, G., & Barris, R. The demystification of health care and demise of the sick role: Implications for occupational therapy. In G. Kielhofner (Ed.), *Health through occupation: Theory and practice in occupational therapy*. Philadelphia: F. A. Davis, 1983.

18. Cantor, S. G. Occupational therapists as members of pre-retirement re-

source teams. *American Journal of Occupational Therapy*, 1981, *35*, 638–643.

19. Carey, C. *Games: An occupational therapy treatment mode for juvenile delinquent boys*. Unpublished master's project, Department of Occupational Therapy, Virginia Commonwealth University, 1981.

20. Casanova, J. S., & Ferber, J. Comprehensive evaluation of basic living skills. *American Journal of Occupational Therapy*, 1976, *30*, 101–105.

21. Corry, S., Sebastian, V., & Mosey, A. C. Acute short-term treatment in psychiatry. *American Journal of Occupational Therapy*, 1974, *28*, 401–406.

22. Cubie, S. H., & Kaplan, K. A case analysis method for the model of human occupation. *American Journal of Occupational Therapy*, 1982, *36*, 645–656.

23. Cynkin, S. *Occupational therapy: Toward health through activities*. Boston: Little, Brown, 1979.

24. Deane, W. N., & Dodd, M. L. Educational techniques for the rehabilitation of chronic schizophrenic patients. *American Journal of Occupational Therapy*, 1960, *14*, 7–12.

25. DeMars, P. K. Training adult retardates for private enterprise. *American Journal of Occupational Therapy*, 1975, *29*, 39–42.

26. deRenne-Stephan, C. Imitation: A mechanism of play behavior. *American Journal of Occupational Therapy*, 1980, *34*, 95–102.

27. Diasio, K. Psychiatric occupational therapy: Search for a conceptual framework in light of psychoanalytic ego psychology and learning theory. *American Journal of Occupational Therapy*, 1968, *22*, 400–414.

28. Dobbins, B. *An investigation of the reliability and validity of the Westphal decision making inventory*. Unpublished master's project, Department of Occupational Therapy, Virginia Commonwealth University, 1980.

29. Donohue, M. V. Designing activities to develop a women's identification group. *Occupational Therapy in Mental Health*, 1982, *2*, 1–19.

30. Dunning, H. Environmental occupational therapy. *American Journal of Occupational Therapy*, 1972, *26*, 292–298.

31. Dunning, R. E. The occupational therapist as counselor. *American Journal of Occupational Therapy*, 1973, *27*, 473–476.

32. Engelhardt, H. T., Jr. Defining occupational therapy: The meaning of therapy and the virtues of occupation. *American Journal of Occupational Therapy*, 1977, *31*, 666–672.

33. Ethridge, D. A. The management view of the future of occupational therapy in mental health. *American Journal of Occupational Therapy*, 1976, *30*, 623–628.

34. Farnham-Diggory, S. Self, future, and time: A developmental study of

the concepts of psychotic, brain-damaged, and normal children. *Monographs of the Society for Research in Child Development*, 1966, *31* (1, Serial No. 103).

35. Fidler, G. Some unique contributions of occupational therapy in the treatment of the schizophrenic. *American Journal of Occupational Therapy*, 1958, *12*, 9–12.

36. Fidler, G. S. The task-oriented group as a context for treatment. *American Journal of Occupational Therapy*, 1969, *23*, 43–48.

37. Fidler, G., & Fidler, J. Doing and becoming: Purposeful action and self-actualization. *American Journal of Occupational Therapy*, 1978, *32*, 305–310.

38. Fidler, G., & Fidler, J. Doing and becoming: The occupational therapy experience. In G. Kielhofner (Ed.), *Health through occupation: Theory and practice in occupational therapy*. Philadelphia: F. A. Davis, 1983.

39. Florey, L. Intrinsic motivation: The dynamics of occupational therapy. *American Journal of Occupational Therapy*, 1969, *23*, 319–322.

40. Florey, L. An approach to play and play development. *American Journal of Occupational Therapy*, 1971, *25*, 275–280.

41. Florey, L., & Michelman, S. Occupational role history: A screening tool for psychiatric occupational therapy. *American Journal of Occupational Therapy*, 1982, *36*, 301–308.

42. Fluegelman, A. (Ed.). *The new games book*. San Francisco: Headlands Press, 1976.

43. Fluegelman, A. *More new games*. Tiburon, Calif.: Headlands Press, 1981.

44. German, S. A. A group approach to rehabilitation occupational therapy in a psychiatric setting. *American Journal of Occupational Therapy*, 1964, *18*, 209–214.

45. Gilfoyle, E. M. Caring: A philosophy for practice. *American Journal of Occupational Therapy*, 1980, *34*, 517–521.

46. Girling, K. L. Leisure counseling. *Canadian Journal of Occupational Therapy*, 1979, *46*, 155–158.

47. Goldstein, N., & Collins, T. Making videotapes: An activity for hospitalized adolescents. *American Journal of Occupational Therapy*, 1982, *36*, 530–533.

48. Goodwin, E. Implementation of the occupational behavior model: A personal account. *Canadian Journal of Occupational Therapy*, 1976, *43*, 14–17.

49. Gray, M. Effects of hospitalization on work-play behavior. *American Journal of Occupational Therapy*, 1972, *26*, 180–185.

50. Gregory, M. *Occupational behavior and life satisfaction among retirees*.

Unpublished master's project, Department of Occupational Therapy, Virginia Commonwealth University, 1981.

51. Hasselkus, B. R. Relocation stress and the elderly. *American Journal of Occupational Therapy*, 1978, *32*, 631–636.

52. Heard, C. Occupational role acquisition: A perspective on the chronically disabled. *American Journal of Occupational Therapy*, 1977, *31*, 243–247.

53. Heine, D. Daily living group: Focus on transition from hospital to community. *American Journal of Occupational Therapy*, 1975, *29*, 628–630.

54. Hofstadter, D. R. *Godel, Escher, Bach: An internal golden braid*. New York: Basic Books, 1979.

55. Howe, M. C., Weaver, C. T., & Dulay, J. The development of a work-oriented day care program. *American Journal of Occupational Therapy*, 1981, *35*, 711–718.

56. Hurff, J. Gaming technique: An assessment and training tool for individuals with learning deficits. *American Journal of Occupational Therapy*, 1981, *35*, 728–735.

57. Kannegieter, R. Environmental interactions in psychiatric occupational therapy—Some inferences. *American Journal of Occupational Therapy*, 1980, *34*, 715–720.

58. Kaplan, K. *Directive group*. Unpublished paper, Department of Occupational Therapy, Virginia Commonwealth University, 1972.

59. Kaseman, B. M. Teaching money management skills to psychiatric outpatients. *Occupational Therapy in Mental Health*, 1980, *1*, 59–71.

60. Kavanaugh, M. *Person-environment interaction: The model of human occupation applied to mentally retarded adults*. Unpublished master's project, Department of Occupational Therapy, Virginia Commonwealth University, 1982.

61. Kielhofner, G. Temporal adaptation: A conceptual framework for occupational therapy. *American Journal of Occupational Therapy*, 1977, *31*, 235–238.

62. Kielhofner, G. A model of human occupation, Part 2. Ontogenesis from the perspective of temporal adaptation. *American Journal of Occupational Therapy*, 1980, *34*, 657–663.

63. Kielhofner, G. A model of human occupation, Part 3. Benign and vicious cycles. *American Journal of Occupational Therapy*, 1980, *34*, 732–737.

64. Kielhofner, G. A paradigm for practice: The hierarchical organization of occupational therapy knowledge. In G. Kielhofner (Ed.), *Health through occupation: Theory and practice in occupational therapy*. Philadelphia: F. A. Davis, 1983.

65. Kielhofner, G., Barris, R., & Watts, J. Habits and habit dysfunction: A

clinical perspective for psychosocial occupational therapy. *Occupational Therapy in Mental Health*, 1982, *2*, 1–22.

66. Kielhofner, G., & Burke, J. P. A model of human occupation, Part 1. Conceptual framework and content. *American Journal of Occupational Therapy*, 1980, *34*, 572–581.

67. Kielhofner, G., & Burke, J. P. The evolution of knowledge and practice in occupational therapy: Past, present and future. In G. Kielhofner (Ed.), *Health through occupation: Theory and practice in occupational therapy*. Philadelphia: F. A. Davis, 1983.

68. Kielhofner, G., Burke, J. P., & Igi, C. H. A model of human occupation, Part 4. Assessment and intervention. *American Journal of Occupational Therapy*, 1980, *34*, 777–788.

69. Kielhofner, G., & Miyake, S. The therapeutic use of games with mentally retarded adults. *American Journal of Occupational Therapy*, 1981, *35*, 375–382.

70. Kielhofner, G., & Miyake, S. Rose-colored lenses for clinical practice: From a deficit to a competence model in assessment and intervention. In G. Kielhofner (Ed.), *Health through occupation: Theory and practice in occupational therapy*. Philadelphia: F. A. Davis, 1983.

71. Kielhofner, G., & Takata, N. A study of mentally retarded persons: Applied research in occupational therapy. *American Journal of Occupational Therapy*, 1980, *34*, 252–258.

72. King, L. J. A sensory-integrative approach to schizophrenia. *American Journal of Occupational Therapy*, 1974, *28*, 529–536.

73. Kirchman, M. M., Reichenbach, V., & Giambalvo, B. Preventive activities and services for the well elderly. *American Journal of Occupational Therapy*, 1982, *36*, 236–242.

74. Klavins, R. Work-play behavior: Cultural influences. *American Journal of Occupational Therapy*, 1972, *26*, 176–179.

75. Kluckholn, F. R., & Strodtbeck, F. L. *Variations in value orientations*. New York: Row, Peterson, 1961.

76. Knox, S. *Observation and assessment of the everyday play behavior of the mentally retarded child*. Unpublished master's thesis, Department of Occupational Therapy, University of Southern California, 1968.

77. Knox, S. A play scale. In M. Reilly (Ed.), *Play as exploratory learning*. Beverly Hills, Calif.: Sage Publications, 1974.

78. Kohler, E. S. The effect of activity/environment on emotionally disturbed children. *American Journal of Occupational Therapy*, 1980, *34*, 446–451.

79. Kolodner, E. L. Neighborhood extension of activity therapy. *American Journal of Occupational Therapy*, 1973, *27*, 381–383.

80. Kuenstler, G. A planning group for psychiatric outpatients. *American Journal of Occupational Therapy*, 1976, *30*, 634–639.
81. Larrington, G. *An exploratory study of the temporal aspects of adaptive functioning.* Unpublished master's thesis, Department of Occupational Therapy, University of Southern California, 1970.
82. Lawn, E. C., & O'Kane, C. P. Psychosocial symbols as communicative media. *American Journal of Occupational Therapy*, 1973, *27*, 30–33.
83. Lerner, C., & Ross, G. The magazine picture collage: Development of an objective scoring system. *American Journal of Occupational Therapy*, 1977, *31*, 156–161.
84. Levin, S. *Test-retest reliability of the Westphal decision making inventory.* Unpublished master's project, Department of Occupational Therapy, Virginia Commonwealth University, 1981.
85. Lillie, M. D., & Armstrong, H. E., Jr. Contributions to the development of psychoeducational approaches to mental health service. *American Journal of Occupational Therapy*, 1982, *36*, 438–443.
86. Lindquist, J., Mack, W., & Parham, D. A synthesis of occupational behavior and sensory integrative concepts in theory and practice, Part 1. Theoretical foundations. *American Journal of Occupational Therapy*, 1982, *36*, 365–374.
87. Lindquist, J., Mack, W., & Parham, D. A synthesis of occupational behavior and sensory integration concepts in theory and practice, Part 2. Clinical applications. *American Journal of Occupational Therapy*, 1982, *36*, 433–437.
88. Linnell, M. W., Caffey, E. M., Klett, C. J., Hogarty, G. E., & Lamb, R. L. Day treatment and psychotropic drugs in the aftercare of schizophrenic patients. *Archives of General Psychiatry*, 1979, *36*, 1055–1066.
• 89. Linnell, K., Stechman, A., & Watson, C. Resocialization of schizophrenic patients. *American Journal of Occupational Therapy*, 1975, *29*, 288–290.
90. Llorens, L. Facilitating growth and development: The promise of occupational therapy. *American Journal of Occupational Therapy*, 1970, *24*, 93–101.
91. Magill, J., & Vargo, J. Helplessness, hope and the occupational therapist. *Canadian Journal of Occupational Therapy*, 1977, *44*, 65–69.
92. Mann, W. C. A quarterway house for adult psychiatric patients. *American Journal of Occupational Therapy*, 1976, *30*, 646–647.
93. Matsutsuyu, J. S. The interest checklist. *American Journal of Occupational Therapy*, 1969, *23*, 323–328.
94. Matsutsuyu, J. Occupational behavior—A perspective on work and play. *American Journal of Occupational Therapy*, 1971, *25*, 291–294.
95. Meacham, R., & Lindemann, J. E. A summer program for underachiev-

ing adolescents. *American Journal of Occupational Therapy*, 1975, *29*, 280–283.

96. Menarcheck, M. *Examining the validity of the play history*. Unpublished master's project, Department of Occupational Therapy, Virginia Commonwealth University, 1982.

97. Michelman, S. Play and the deficit child. In M. Reilly (Ed.), *Play as exploratory learning*. Beverly Hills, Calif.: Sage Publications, 1974.

98. Moorhead, L. The occupational history. *American Journal of Occupational Therapy*, 1969, *23*, 329–334.

99. Mosey, A. Recapitulation of ontogenesis: A theory for practice of occupational therapy. *American Journal of Occupational Therapy*, 1968, *22*, 426–438.

100. Mosey, A. C. The concept and use of developmental groups. *American Journal of Occupational Therapy*, 1970, *24*, 272–275.

101. Mosey, A. C. *Occupational therapy: Configuration of a profession*. New York: Raven Press, 1981.

102. Neville, A. Temporal adaptation: Application with short-term psychiatric patients. *American Journal of Occupational Therapy*, 1980, *34*, 328–331.

103. Nihara, K., Foster, R., Shellhaas, M., & Leland, H. *AAMD Adaptive Behavior Scale*. Washington, D.C.: American Association on Mental Deficiency, 1974.

104. Nystrom, E. P. Activity patterns and leisure concepts among the elderly. *American Journal of Occupational Therapy*, 1974, *28*, 337–345.

105. Oakley, F. M. *The model of human occupation in psychiatry*. Unpublished master's project, Department of Occupational Therapy, Virginia Commonwelath University, 1982.

106. Parent, L. Effects of a low-stimulus environment on behavior. *American Journal of Occupational Therapy*, 1978, *32*, 19–25.

107. Paulson, C. Juvenile delinquency and occupational choice. *American Journal of Occupational Therapy*, 1980, *34*, 565–571.

108. Potts, L. *Toward a developmental assessment of leisure patterns*. Unpublished master's thesis, Department of Occupational Therapy, University of Southern California, 1969.

109. Reilly, M. Occupational therapy can be one of the great ideas of 20th century medicine. *American Journal of Occupational Therapy*, 1962, *16*, 1–9.

110. Reilly, M. A. A psychiatric occupational therapy program as a teaching model. *American Journal of Occupational Therapy*, 1966, *20*, 61–67.

111. Reilly, M. *Play as exploratory learning*. Beverly Hills, Calif.: Sage Publications, 1974.

112. Riopel, N. J. *An examination of the occupational behavior and life satis-faction of the elderly.* Unpublished master's thesis, Medical College of Virginia, Virginia Commonwealth University, 1982.

113. Robinson, A. Play: The arena for acquisition of rules for competent behavior. *American Journal of Occupational Therapy*, 1977, *31*, 248–253.

114. Rogers, J. Order and disorder in medicine and occupational therapy. *American Journal of Occupational Therapy*, 1982, *36*, 29–35.

115. Rogers, J. C., & Snow, T. An assessment of the behaviors of the institutionalized elderly. *American Journal of Occupational Therapy*, 1982, *36*, 375–380.

116. Rogers, J., Weinstein, J., & Figone, J. An empirical assessment of the interest checklist. *American Journal of Occupational Therapy*, 1978.

117. Roos, P., & Albers, R. Performance of retardates and normals on a measure of temporal orientation. *American Journal of Mental Deficiency*, 1965, *69*, 835–838.

118. Rotter, J. Generalized expectancies for internal versus external control for reinforcement. *Psychological Monographs*, 1966, *80* (1, Whole No. 609).

119. Scaffa, M. *Temporal adaptation and alcoholism.* Unpublished master's project, Department of Occupational Therapy, Virginia Commonwealth University, 1981.

120. Scheflen, A. E. *Body language and social order.* Englewood Cliffs, N. J.: Prentice-Hall, 1972.

121. Shannon, P. Work-play theory and the occupational therapy process. *American Journal of Occupational Therapy*, 1972, *26*, 169–172.

122. Shannon, P. Occupational choice: Decision making play. In M. Reilly (Ed.), *Play as exploratory learning.* Beverly Hills, Calif.: Sage Publications, 1974.

123. Sharrott, G. Occupational therapy's role in the client's creation and affirmation of meaning. In G. Kielhofner (Ed.), *Health through occupation: Theory and practice in occupational therapy.* Philadelphia: F. A. Davis, 1983.

124. Shroeder, C. V., Block, M. P., Trottier, & Stowell, M. S. The adult psychiatric sensory integrative evaluation. In B. Hemphill (Ed.), *The evaluative process in psychiatric occupational therapy.* Thoroughfare, N. J.: Charles B. Slack, 1982.

125. Takata, N. Play as a prescription. In M. Reilly (Ed.), *Play as exploratory learning.* Beverly Hills, Calif.: Sage Publications, 1974.

126. Vandenberg, B., & Kielhofner, G. Play in evolution, culture and individual adaptation: Implications for therapy. *American Journal of Occupational Therapy*, 1982, *36*, 20–28.

127. Versluys, H. P. The remediation of role disorders through focused group work. *American Journal of Occupational Therapy*, 1980, *34*, 609–614.

128. Watts, J., & Barris, R. *Aging Person-environment interaction and the model of human occupation*. Richmond: Virginia Commonwealth University, 1981. (Audiovisual production)

129. Watanabe, S. Four concepts to the occupational therapy process. *American Journal of Occupational Therapy*, 1968, *22*, 339–444.

130. Webb, L. J. The therapeutic social club. *American Journal of Occupational Therapy*, 1973, *27*, 81–83.

131. Webster, P. Occupational role development in the young adult with mild mental retardation. *American Journal of Occupational Therapy*, 1980, *34*, 13–18.

132. Wiemer, R. Traditional and nontraditional practice arenas. In *Occupational therapy: 2001 A.D.* Rockville, Md.: American Occupational Therapy Association, 1979.

133. Westphal, M. *A study of decision making*. Unpublished master's thesis, Department of Occupational Therapy, University of Southern California, 1967.

134. Yerxa, E. Occupational therapy's role in creating a future climate of caring. *American Journal of Occupational Therapy*, 1980, *34*, 529–534.

5

Criticisms and Limitations

The most obvious limitation of the occupational therapy tradition in psychosocial practice is the one that has been emphasized throughout this volume. Occupational therapy practice in the area of psychosocial dysfunction has a very specific and therefore circumscribed purpose and intent: to improve people's capacity for and involvement in healthy occupations. As such, it does not address some of the problems inherent in psychosocial dysfunction. Interestingly, therapists have not always recognized or agreed to these limits. For example, the whole domain of sexual feelings and unconscious processes are beyond the scope of occupational therapy, yet many therapists have made these issues focal points of their practice.

In addition, since occupational therapy focuses on the maintenance and development of healthy behavior, it has limited relevance to many aspects of psychopathology as conceptualized by the medical model. Reilly[4] suggested that occupational therapy makes no claim to influence pathological states; however, this issue bears further exploration. Occupational therapy has limited impact on pathology in terms of psychiatric diagnostic categories. That is, it is not directed at influencing any psychodynamics underlying such states as anorexia or modifying symptomatic events such as hallucinations. Other contributions in the mental health arena such as psychotherapy and chemotherapy do make claims to have an influence on such pathological phenomena.

On the other hand, because psychosocial dysfunction frequently involves the interplay of several etiological and syndromatic factors—some of which may be occupational in nature—a program of occupational therapy aimed at influencing healthy occupational behavior could have some impact on pathological processes. The limitation of occupational therapy is that it does not specifically seek to remediate pathology. For example, occupational therapy, with its concentration on life tasks and concrete performance, may increase the reality-based thinking of the schizophrenic patient. Or because of its emphasis on eliciting feelings of competence and control, it may reduce symptoms of clinical depression or the anxiety level of a psychotic person. But even in such cases, the goal of treatment is not symptom reduction. Thus, while the contribution of occupational therapists to influencing pathology is limited, it nonetheless may exist as an indirect result of therapy.

This is not to suggest that occupational therapy has a more limited contribution than other disciplines to make to those with psychosocial problems. On the contrary, occupational problems are part and parcel of psychosocial disorder, and the occupational therapist is in a special position to address and ameliorate such problems.

The process of setting limits on what one does as a professional is a critical one, lest a field be accused of claiming to be "all things to all people." At times in the past, occupational therapists have come dangerously close to this or have actually made such claims, attempting to use occupational media for any purpose they chose. All fields and their respective views of order and disorder, along with their action implications, offer only partial answers to complex psychosocial problems. Each is limited by its particular focus and expertise.

Another important limitation of occupational therapy is the "state of the art." As a relatively new field that has placed less emphasis on developing a coherent body of knowledge than on refining practical techniques, the field has less sophisticated concepts and fewer connections between theory and practice than fields such as behavioral psychology that have stressed science as much as practical application. The manifestations of this limitation are: (1) the lack of conceptual refinement of theory (especially refinement based on research); (2) the preliminary nature of most clinical assessments (i.e., most lack research claims to reliability and validity); (3) the limited connections between theory and practice (i.e., many theoretical formulations do not have clearly articulated action principles, and many practical programs described in the literature are not firmly based in theory); and (4) the lack of outcome research on practice techniques and programs.

Another limitation of occupational therapy is the degree to which most occupational therapists understand the main tradition and themes of the field. Over the years therapists in a variety of settings have come under pressure to accept and apply the knowledge of traditions other than occupational therapy. For example, one can find occupational therapy programs based primarily on behavioral or psychoanalytic concepts. Such programs not only obscure the uniqueness of occupational therapy, but they limit the contribution that clinical practice could otherwise make to the development of technologies of practice for the field. Because the perspective offered in this volume on occupational therapy practice is not at present universally accepted, disagreement, dialogue, and eventual consensus will have to occur before clear and concentrated development of the knowledge and practice base can take place. In this vein, Bockoven[1,2] has criticized occupational therapy for its lack of recognition of its moral mandate and its inattention to the mental problems of disordered society (i.e., poor conditions of work and play that lead to psychosocial dysfunction). Bockoven is referring to the fact that occupational therapy has often taken the route of existing psychodynamic or other approaches, rather than developing and pursuing its own unique contribution to psychosocial health.

It could be said that occupational therapy's historical mandate is certainly much larger than that which has already been realized in clinical practice. Reilly[3] saw occupational therapy as being one of the great ideas of 20th century medicine, yet its practice does not reflect such importance. This is both discouraging, since it indicates that the field has been slow to operationalize its hypothesis that occupation can influence health, and encouraging, since it points to a great potential for the field if efforts are consolidated to advance theory, research, and practice.

A criticism that occupational therapists in practice will be familiar with is one that comes from other professionals as they view occupational therapy in psychosocial treatment. That is, the practical focus of the field, its concern for playful media and the like, is often misinterpreted by other disciplines as a sign that occupational therapy is not an important therapy or that it is primarily diversional in nature. In other words, it keeps patients busy but doesn't really have any impact on their problems.

In the past it is this criticism that appears to have led therapists to abandon their orientation and their occupational media in favor of assuming roles more like those of others in the setting—for example, running verbal groups with no occupational component. Therapists should recognize that such criticism is not founded in an objective analysis of occupational therapy but in misunderstanding. As Reilly[3] once noted, the vast difference between the complexity of our patient problems and the very simple media we use to address those problems is both our greatest asset and our greatest vulnerability. Therapists should seek ways to translate criticism into a recognition of occupational therapy as an asset. Inservice education and clearly formulated and theoretically based program descriptions are examples of the kinds of tools that therapists can use to explain their therapy, its goals, and how it works.

REFERENCES

1. Bockoven, J. S. Challenge of the new clinical approaches. *American Journal of Occupational Therapy*, 1968, *22*, 23–25.
2. Bockoven, J. S. *Moral treatment in community mental health.* New York: Springer Publishing, 1972.

3. Reilly, M. Occupational therapy can be one of the great ideas of 20th century medicine. *American Journal of Occupational Therapy*, 1983, *16*, 1–9.
4. Reilly, M. A psychiatric occupational therapy program as a teaching model. *American Journal of Occupational Therapy*, 1966, *20*, 61–67.

6

Commentary

In proposing a unique occupational therapy approach to psychosocial practice, this book showed how certain themes and principles have emerged and been enacted by therapists. These themes capture what we perceive to be the longstanding central tradition of the field, and they provide a cohesive framework for delineating the role of occupational therapy in psychosocial practice.

Some will no doubt view our concentration on occupation and occupational dysfunction and our relative exclusion of such concepts and approaches such as psychoanalytically based occupational therapy as unnecessarily confining to both the scholarship and practice of occupational therapy. We are the first to acknowledge that our approach definitively sets limits on the boundaries of occupational therapy's expertise and defines the nature of its practice in a narrower sense than others have proposed.

It is not the intention of this volume to limit occupational therapists' awareness of a wide range of knowledge. For this reason we authored another volume, *Bodies of Knowledge in Psychosocial Practice*, which covers major theoretical perspectives in psychosocial practice today. However, we do reject the notion that all this knowledge should be treated equally by occupational therapists. Occupational therapists must evaluate and determine what any knowledge has to offer their practice by selecting judiciously that which is complementary and leaving out that which is not necessary or relevant. To fail to do so perpetuates ambiguity in psychosocial occupational therapy practice and results in the inability of the field to either define its special area of expertise or to admit limitations in the range of competencies of its practitioners. In the past such failure has diluted occupational therapists' grasp of what they should uniquely know how to do and obscured the identity that would make occupational therapists valuable and definable members of a psychosocial health care team.

The dilution of the occupational therapist's knowledge and identity that has resulted from an eclectic, broad-based approach to psychosocial practice can actually be more limiting in the long run. Therapists who try to embrace all theories eventually find that their practices reflect the expectations or needs of other professionals, often at the expense of their own beliefs. On the other hand, therapists who identify with a unique theoretical tradition that gives a focus to their role are in a better position to define what services they have to offer and then to competently provide them. Rather than confining, a unique professional theory allows the practitioner to understand pluralistic viewpoints without losing sight of his or her own perspective.

The focus on occupation that we have identified as central to occupational therapy is far from being a restrictive perspective for the field. Occupation is a complex phenomenon that can take us to a wide range of concerns and studies. Within this general rubric there is ample room for creativity, diversity of thought, and variety of research, theory, and practice. Even more important, the focus on occupation reflects the historical mandate of the field as well as mainstream beliefs and principles of occupational therapists practicing in psychosocial settings today. Belief in the occupational nature of people and a treatment emphasis on work, play, and self-care continues to characterize the practice of many occupational therapists and, in particular, that of therapists who are most likely to think and act as autonomous professionals.[1]

Hence, it is not only *not* confining to set limits on the scope of practice, but it can serve to strengthen and ensure the professional survival of the field. In fact, it is probably unwise to seek survival by trying to fit in and adopt the ideas of others, because the health care system of today is itself in a state of flux.

For instance, such trends as increasing concern over cost-effectiveness, the movement of health care into the private corporate sector, and the growing awareness and power of the consumer who wants to be informed will increasingly make demands on occupational therapy to clearly articulate its service and the benefits of that service. At the same time that such changes in health care will call for a more clearly delineated service, there will be changes that would welcome the kind of occupational therapy service we have articulated in this book. As consumers become more aware that health is a matter of what they do, they will be looking for health care that supports their doing instead of simply repairing their deficits. Health care in general is recognizing that health is a state greatly influenced by the person's daily action and interaction with the environment. A service model which provides opportunity for active involvement and which addresses the process of every-day competence will flourish in such an arena.

While the system is changing, we are well aware that the present health care system has created many impediments to our practice. Issues of reim-bursability for our services and gaining recognition from other psychosocial workers can be major obstacles, but they are not insurmountable. In fact, some of the difficulty we currently face in obtaining third-party reimbursement for occupational goals and means has resulted because we did not have a clear sense of our mission in the past and others defined for us what should be reimbursed. Shaping practice to what we can get paid for, rather than to what individuals really need, may allow us to survive in the short run, but in the long run it will fail because we will no longer be maintaining the social contract that initiated the field's existence.

Like all fields, occupational therapy came into existence and initially gained financial and social support from society because it served an identifiable need. This need was for reality-based programs of occupation that could reorient and rehabilitate disabled persons. As we have strayed from this historical mandate, other fields have quickly stepped in to fill the gap, so obviously the need for the type of service we can offer still exists.

Given both the historical reasons for the emergence of occupational therapy and the current changes in the health care system, occupational therapy can hardly afford to remain an ambiguous service, unsure of its unique contri-bution in health care. While identifying with the knowledge and techniques of other professions or blending into the philosophies of particular settings may be a path of least resistance or a means of gaining acceptance or respect for individual therapists in the short run, it would be professional suicide in the long run.

Having a viable practice requires a unified professional identity. The source of such an identity and practice is already available in the field's tradition of knowledge. This book should be a step toward enhancing the identification and operationalization of a unique and unified occupational therapy service.

REFERENCE

1. Barris, R. *Toward an image of one's own: Sources of variation in the oc-cupational therapist's role.* Unpublished doctoral dissertation, Teacher's College, Columbia University, New York, 1983.